Smart Lotionmaking
The Simple Guide to Making Luxurious Lotions

— Anne L. Watson —

Anne L. Watson's *Smart Soapmaking* was the first book based on modern techniques that eliminate the drudgery and guesswork from home soapmaking. Now, by popular demand, she continues her handcraft cosmetics revolution with the first practical, comprehensive book on making lotion.

Whether you want to make lotion for personal use or to sell, Anne allays any fears with methods that are proven safe and approved by experts, yet simple and easy enough to perform in your kitchen. You'll soon be making lotion that's better than any you've been buying, and at a fraction of the cost.

"The definitive guide to lotionmaking."

Donna Puizina, Ekoaromas
Lafayette, New Jersey

"Spells out everything and makes it easy to understand."

Cheryl McCoy, Emerald City Soap
Haven, Kansas

"Anne makes it so much fun, and so easy."

Mary Jean Hammann
Grandma Jean's Soaps and Lotions
New London, Ohio

"So logical and easy to understand that my first batch was a success *and* a sell-out!"

Susan Dinion, Holiday Farm
Berlin, Massachusetts

BOOKS BY ANNE L. WATSON

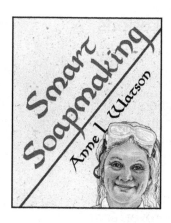

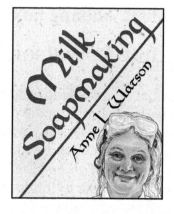

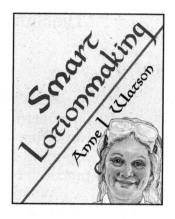

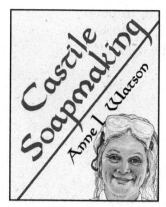

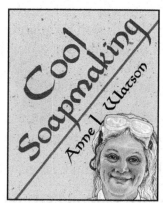

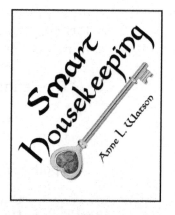

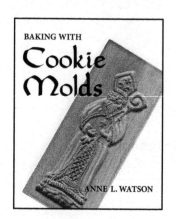

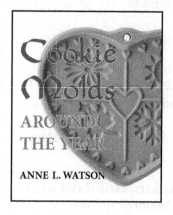

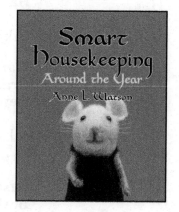

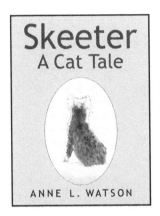

Skeeter
A Cat Tale
ANNE L. WATSON

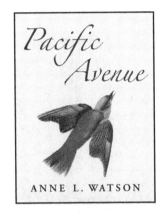

Pacific Avenue
ANNE L. WATSON

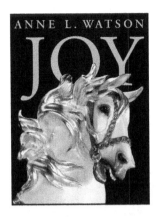

ANNE L. WATSON
JOY

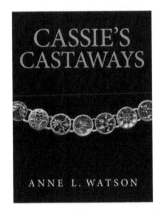

CASSIE'S CASTAWAYS
ANNE L. WATSON

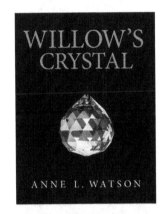

WILLOW'S CRYSTAL
ANNE L. WATSON

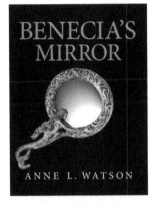

BENECIA'S MIRROR
ANNE L. WATSON

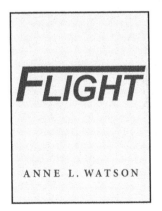

FLIGHT
ANNE L. WATSON

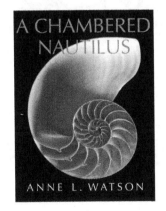

A CHAMBERED NAUTILUS
ANNE L. WATSON

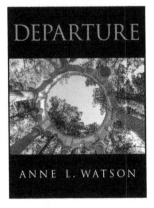

DEPARTURE
ANNE L. WATSON

and more . . .

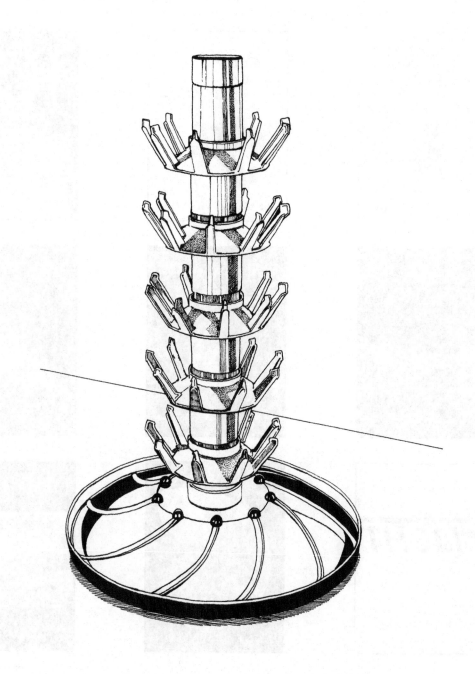

Smart Lotionmaking

The Simple Guide to Making Luxurious Lotions

OR

How to Make Lotion That's Better Than You Buy and Costs You Less

Anne L. Watson

Illustrated by Wendy Edelson

Shepard Publications
Friday Harbor, Washington

Back cover photo by Aaron Shepard, with lotions courtesy of Linda
Francis, Friday Harbor, Washington

Version 1.2

To the Soap Sisters

Contents

Acknowledgments

I'd like to thank my testers and commenters, who tried lotions and recipes, reviewed and used my manuscript, and provided invaluable opinions and suggestions: Yvonne Bowman, Tina Marie Carelli, Liz Cifani, Ingrid DeBree, Susanna Dinion, Laurie Drake, Kevin M. Dunn, Linda Francis, Maria M. Gonzalez, Amanda Guilfoyle, Pip Guyatt, Mary Jean Hammann, Carol Holt, Terry Holt, Deena Humphrey, Cindy Jones, Susan Kennedy, Ruth Kohl, Christine Mays, Cheryl McCoy, Loretta McPherson, Tricia Miller, Lydia Nelson, Pat Potter, Marge Robbins, Dawn Robnett, Gail Schnee, Randy Schnee, Beth Signor, Marilyn Smith, Mary Sonier, Louise Sturdivant, Tami Thornton, Becky Utecht, Kaci Waller, and Sandy Wilson.

Additional thanks to those who contributed guest recipes: Ingrid DeBree, Linda Francis, Amanda Guilfoyle, Deena Humphrey, and Susan Kennedy.

Special thanks to Linda Francis, whose shared knowledge of microbiology was so essential to my exploration of lotionmaking.

To biochemist Neil Dobson, for invaluable information concerning formulating and other lotionmaking matters.

To my husband, Aaron Shepard, for editing, book design, and general coordination.

To Kathy Ford, who taught me to make lotion, and never so much as suggested there was anything hard about it.

A Few First Thoughts

I have no idea why anyone would *buy* lotion. It's a mystery.

Maybe it's because of *another* mystery: the lotions themselves. With even halfway decent lotions so expensive, they must somehow be hard to make, right?

Not really. If we all knew how easy it was to make our own lotion, the stores could clear a lot of shelf space. Who would buy what they could make better, and at a tenth of the cost?

The thing is, few people believe that lotionmaking *could* be easy—not before they've tried it, that is.

It seems like it would *have* to be hard. It's hard to even read the ingredients, when you look at consumer labels. By the time you've plowed through methylparaben, triethanolamine, butylene glycol, glycol stearate, glyceryl stearate, disodium EDTA, aluminum magnesium silicate, DMDM hydantoin, and tocopheryl acetate, you're just about ready to give up—and if that doesn't do it, you'll definitely throw up your hands at 3-iodo-2-propynylbutylcarbamate. You wouldn't know where to *get* that stuff, much less what to do with it once you did.

Honey, I'm running to the store for DMDM hydantoin and 3-iodo-2-propynylbutylcarbamate. Anything you need while I'm out?

But, whatever manufacturers do to make bottles of lotion by the millions, handcraft lotionmaking is much simpler. It's a lot like making salad dressing. Of course, if you make lotion to sell, it will be regulated by law, just like food in a restaurant—but making it for your own use is like cooking at home. You'll work clean, as you would for cooking, but you won't be held to commercial standards.

I'll show you how to make lotion for yourself in a way that's clean *enough*—and how to check if that causes any problem. It isn't likely to. I've made lotion for myself for years, and never had any go bad.

In some cases, you should sanitize more thoroughly. So, this book will give two different methods for making lotion. *Personal Technique* is for simple lotion meant for your own use. This one is quicker and easier. *Pro Technique* is for lotion you mean to sell, or for lotion with perishable ingredients like milk, or for lotion with no preservative. This one isn't difficult either—just more painstaking and precise.

But why the difference? After all, you wouldn't want something insanitary for your own use. Why wouldn't you follow the same procedure for any lotion?

The answer is that Pro Technique is designed to conform to common laws and regulations for commercial lotionmaking. These laws and regulations have to address almost anything that can happen. They have to prevent the sale of lotion made in filthy conditions by people who have no idea what they're doing. They have to apply the same way to everyone. And with all that, they're simply more than you need for most home use.

Still, the difference between the techniques isn't huge. And whichever you try, you'll soon be making lotion better than you're likely to find at any price.

Lies and Lotions
Myths About Lotion and Lotionmaking

There are a number of serious misconceptions about lotion and lotionmaking. Let's take time to discuss them—because even if they don't quite scare you away, they'll slow you down.

Myth #1: Making lotion is difficult.

I was lucky—I didn't hear this one till I knew better. The first time someone asked in an awed tone if I'd really made lotion, I was surprised. But many people don't make things at all and are amazed by those who do—so I didn't think much about it.

But the first time a *soapmaker* asked that same question, and in that same tone, I was truly puzzled. Heaven knows, soap is easy enough to make, but lotion is still easier. Why would a soapmaker be impressed by handmade lotion?

Thinking it over, I decided it made sense of a sort. Regardless of the chemical stew I described earlier, if you read the label on even a bottle of natural lotion, you'll find it's mostly water—and the rest is mostly oils. No great expense there. So you might then figure that the high price reflects the difficulty of making the lotion.

But you'd guess wrong. Though it's possible to make a lotion that would disappoint you, a complete failure would be very rare. So why are even halfway decent lotions such upmarket items?

Part of it may be meeting commercial sanitation require-ments in an industrial setting. But the rest is packaging, ship-ping, insurance, advertising, middlemen, and profit. In other words, you're paying a lot for someone to do what you could do yourself—and easily.

Myth #2: Making lotion is expensive.

You do need a little gear—but if you cook, you probably have most of it already. And even if you don't, the things you need to get started aren't expensive.

For large-scale commercial lotionmaking, you'd probably want restaurant equipment—good value for money, but not cheap. But by the time you're making dozens of bottles of lotion at once, I'd assume you'd be ready to invest in that.

As for the ingredients, they're not expensive. Even luxury oils don't add up to a big expense in making lotion. When your product is 80% water, you can put in some pretty fancy stuff without breaking the bank.

And here's a little-known fact: Some common ingredients are actually *better* than luxury ones. I'll discuss that when we talk about designing your own recipes.

To tell the truth, one of the most important "ingredients" isn't an ingredient at all: It's regular use. When I started this book, I was an on-again, off-again lotion user with minor but persistent dry skin problems—rough hands and feet, mostly. Making and testing dozens of lotions, putting them on my hands and feet daily, I soon got to where I had to find other testers. That's because I could no longer tell much about any one lotion—my skin was in too good shape to improve much.

I hadn't used one "miracle" product. In fact, I hadn't used any of my lotions more than a few times. The important thing wasn't any exotic ingredient. It was just using good lotion daily.

Myth #3: Lotion you make yourself isn't going to be very good.

I think this one got started with the easy availability of pre-made lotion base. If you go to a soapmaker's booth at the farmers' market, the soap will be handmade. But all too often, the lotion is treated as only a sideline, and will be made from a purchased base with scent added.

I did a great deal of testing in the course of writing this book, sending little bottles of lotion to testers all over. They had no idea what was in the bottles, since each was identified only by a number. Unknown to my testers, I threw in a few ringers—lotions made from kits, plus one with a pre-made commercial base.

There was no lotion that pleased everyone, but there was one that almost everyone disliked. You guessed it. It was the one with the commercial base.

What's especially interesting is they disliked it for different reasons.

> *"It soaked in fast, but I needed more in just a short time."*

> *"Felt sticky for almost an hour."*

> *"I keep putting it on, and it sinks in quickly. In fact, it disappears. It's like I never used anything at all."*

So, if you haven't been impressed by "handmade" lotion, maybe you haven't tried the real thing.

Learn how to design a lotion, and experiment with different formulations. Probably some won't work as well as others on your skin—but with a little experimenting, you're likely to find something you'd pay serious money for.

Isn't it nice you won't have to?

Myth #4: Making lotion requires a lot of technical knowledge.

Back to those samples I sent to my testers. The kit lotions had about a 50-50 rating. About half the testers liked them, and some of those liked them a lot.

> *"I'm addicted to that Lotion #1. It's exactly what I needed."*

But the rest gave negative reviews—*really* negative.

> *"Lotion #1 is so greasy, I guess I could use it on my feet, but that's about it."*

That worried me. Those were expensive, top-of-the-line kits from some of the best vendors in the United States. And as I've already said, I got a nearly universal thumbs-down for commercially prepared lotion base. If that was the best the pros could do, it seemed pretty nervy of me to hope to do better.

But I did have the recipe for a lotion I'd made successfully for myself for many years. I had no idea where it came from originally, and neither did the friend who gave it to me.

I studied the proportions and tried a few similar recipes. I learned about the oils and butters that go into lotions—mostly by reading what massage therapists have to say. Now, *those* are people who *really* care how various oils feel. They have to. They spend their days with those oils on their hands, and they won't get much repeat business if their clients go home feeling like greased pigs.

My study got sidetracked for a while by the technicalities of emulsifiers. But I finally realized that several easily available emulsifiers are just fine without any tinkering.

So, I put together some lotions I hoped might work, and sent them to my testers.

What I got back from them was confusion—but a pleasant kind. Many were unsure how to rate the lotions I'd formulated, because they liked them all! There were suggestions—mostly about making the first ones a little thinner. Because the lotions were unscented, the testers noticed the scent of the ingredients themselves, and some didn't care for that. But most of the lotions I designed were quite successful.

Here are a few of the comments:

> *"One thing I did notice in general: They really work! With store-bought lotions, even my favorite, I would have to reapply just about every time I washed my hands. Now I go two or three hand washes before my hands feel like they need lotion."*

> *"I think all of the lotions are good. There is something special about #17. It feels like whipped cream, going on. For about five minutes, it feels like it could be greasy, but then it moisturizes and sinks into my skin with no greasy feeling. It is amazing."*

> *"I love the texture of all of them, smooth and creamy and not too thin. None of them are greasy."*

I'm not kidding myself that I'm an inspired professional formulator. I'm just saying you don't have to be.

Myth #5: Lotion has to be sterile.

I was surprised to learn that *sanitary* and *sterile* don't mean the same. *Sterile* is what you need when doing surgery. *All* bacteria, molds, and viruses must be killed.

Sanitary is less extreme. It means that the number of microorganisms is kept relatively low. You *do* need to make lotion under conditions that are sanitary. But, no, you don't need to make anything sterile.

Having learned this, though, I was still utterly confused as to exactly what *sanitary* is and how to get there. I had a million questions. So, I hired a microbiologist to consult on this book, and I'll share much of what I learned from her.

The two methods I'll describe for lotionmaking—Personal Technique and Pro Technique—are for two levels of sanitizing. The first will make sense for most lotion for personal use. The second is for if you sell lotion, or make it with perishable ingredients, or leave out preservative.

Myth #6: Lotion is hard to emulsify.

Maybe it was, back when your grandmother made her own cold cream with beeswax and borax. She probably stirred it by hand, too, wishing there was a better way.

She got her wish. Now, with emulsifiers made just for handmade lotions, I'm not sure you could keep a lotion from emulsifying if you wanted to. It takes no more than two minutes, if that.

You'll read that it's important to combine the ingredients gradually, as you would for mayonnaise. I never do. I just pour them together, mix well, and I'm done. Why do it the hard way?

Myth #7: Lotion should sink in quickly.

When you rub on lotion, your skin will normally absorb it to a point, then resist further penetration. No one likes a lotion that just sits on the skin and feels greasy. On the other hand, if you didn't need a barrier between yourself and the outside world, you wouldn't *have* skin.

You might have second thoughts about using an additive that forces oils deeper into your skin than they would naturally go. Second thoughts or no, I went ahead and tested a lotion with one of these additives—isopropyl myristate, or IPM. At least on my skin, that lotion didn't moisturize more than any of my other formulations, and it didn't sink in quicker. What's more, I was turned off to discover that IPM is used to kill head lice. I won't tell you what you can and can't put in your own formulations, but that additive isn't in mine.

My lotions *will* sink into your skin—but some of them take a few seconds, and you may find that a small amount of lotion is enough. If that's not what you're hoping for, there are other formulations that are absorbed more quickly. My testers differed on which kind they preferred.

If you're selling lotion, try to educate your customers: *Use just a little. Wait just a minute.* They're used to watery commercial lotions. Once they get the idea, they'll probably prefer the slower kind.

Myth #8: Lotion should match your skin pH.

This one got started as a sales pitch. *Pay more for our product, because we match the pH of your skin, and our competitors don't.*

Obviously, you don't want to put anything very acidic or very caustic on your skin. But with anything in a reasonable range, your skin quickly adjusts and returns to normal pH.

There may well be those whose skin is sensitive enough that they have to pay attention to lotion pH. I'm not a dermatologist, and I can't give the advice of one. But in general, skin balances itself.

That doesn't mean you should ignore pH entirely. Your preservative may come with an ideal pH recommended for its working, and you may have trouble if your lotion pH falls too far from it.

Myth #9: Lotion should be free of preservative.

Many people become interested in making lotion because they want to avoid the preservatives in commercial ones.

I'm not a biochemist, so I can't pronounce on whether any particular preservative applied only to your skin is bad for you or not. But preservatives are not all identical chemically—so if you don't trust one, you may find another that seems safer. There are even preservatives sold as natural products. But whatever preservative you're considering—natural or artificial—I recommend that you seek out unbiased test results to help you decide.

If you choose to go preservative-free, I recommend you use Pro Technique as described in this book, make small batches, keep the lotion refrigerated, and not hold onto it for more than about ten days. As for selling such lotion, it's not explicitly illegal—at least in most areas—but it may not be wise. Legal interpretation of terms like "adulterated" and "misbranded" can be stretched quite far on occasion, and you don't want to fall within their reach. Also, your insurer may not cover such products—some do and some don't.

This issue is very controversial, and beyond the scope of this book to resolve. All my own formulations include preservative, so you'll know how much to use if you choose to. But with the caveats above, you can also omit it. Or you can substitute your own choice of preservative, following the manufacturer's directions.

Myth #10: A good lotion works for anyone.

Since skin varies from one person to another, you'll find that each will prefer certain ingredients or proportions. That's only to be expected.

The testers for this book certainly had their favorites. I wish I could say they all liked the same lotion, the most wonderful lotion in the world, the only one you need to try.

It didn't turn out that way. Among the lotions I formulated myself, all were liked by *most* testers—but not a single lotion worked for them all.

Depending on the climate where they lived, the type of work they did, and their skin type, they gave the lotions differing reviews, and sometimes conflicting ones. Some preferred their lotion very light, with minimal moisturizing. Others wanted something heavy—almost a cream.

So, you'll have to experiment to find the kind that works best for you. And if you're making lotion for sale, you should probably make more than one kind and see what suits your customers.

Lotion Lingo
Learning the Jargon

A good way to avoid being completely put off by a subject is to start off by learning its language. And lotionmaking has a few terms you probably don't use much in ordinary conversation.

Luckily, there really are only a few. Let's take a look at them now to avoid confusion as we go along.

Emulsion

Everyone knows that oil and water don't mix. However, you can *force* them to mix. That gives you an *emulsion*. Common examples are mayonnaise and thick salad dressing.

To mix oil and water and *keep* them mixed, you need an *emulsifier*. In mayonnaise, it's egg yolk. In traditional lotionmaking, it was beeswax. Now there are newer emulsifiers—though some lotionmakers still prefer beeswax.

An emulsion can be either water suspended in oil, or oil suspended in water. What basic kind of emulsion you have depends on the ingredient doing the suspending. Lotions, for instance, are always *water emulsions*—oil suspended in water. Other cosmetic emulsions, like creams and ointments, are oil-based.

Selecting and balancing emulsifiers can get fairly technical, and there are sophisticated methods for it. Since this book is for handcraft lotionmakers, including beginners, most of the recipes in this book use one or both of two commonly available emulsifiers—emulsifying wax and conditioning emulsifier.

If your interest leads you further into the chemistry of emulsifiers and professional lotion formulation, you can find a variety of books on the subject of "cosmetic chemistry."

Formulation

The technical term for the composition of a cosmetic emulsion is *formulation*. Many handcraft lotionmakers, though, might be more comfortable calling it a *recipe*. I don't think there's any confusion about the meaning of either, so I use both.

Depending on its formulation, a cosmetic emulsion may be described as face lotion, night lotion, hand lotion, body lotion, eye cream, foot cream, or for all I know, left pinky lotion. Aside from marketing claims, there can be real differences among many of these types.

First, as I said, a *lotion* is an oil-in-water emulsion—though the water may come in the form of a water-based liquid such as milk. Typically, lotion is at least 70% water. A *cream* is typically between 20% and 50% water, while an emulsion that's less than 20% water is an *ointment*.

The consistency of lotion varies greatly, from fairly heavy and cream-like, to very light. This depends partly on water content, partly on choice of oils and butters, and partly on choice of emulsifier.

Different consistencies are better for different uses. Hand lotions tend to be thick, especially if they're for winter use in cold climates. Body lotions are usually thinner, and may be formulated with fats that are lighter and more easily absorbed.

Most face lotions for nighttime are actually creams. Face lotions for daytime are usually thin, quick-absorbing, but still moisturizing. Often, lotions of this kind are used under makeup as a base. Ingredients may be chosen for supposed anti-aging qualities, or to avoid clogging pores. Commercial lotions for use near the eyes may be thinner, because of the delicacy of the skin there. Many people prefer face lotions to be unscented.

Phase

To make a lotion, you'll first mix the fats and oil-soluble ingredients together, then you'll mix the water and water-soluble ingredients together, and then you'll combine them. Each of these two basic sets of ingredients—oil-based and water-based—is called a *phase*. So, you have an *oil phase* and a *water phase*.

A third phase consists of ingredients added *after* the oil and water have been emulsified. Typically, these ingredients include preservative and scent. As in this book, this is often called the *cool down phase*.

Some recipes and kits use letters or numbers for the three phases—A, B, C, or 1, 2, 3. But they're still the same phases, no matter what they're called.

Sanitize

Sanitize is different from *sterilize*. To truly *sterilize* every-thing—wipe out all microorganisms, as a hospital would do for surgery—is impossible in handcraft lotionmaking. Instead, you'll *sanitize*—reduce the level of microorganisms to a rea-sonably safe level.

If you're making lotion only for yourself, the extent of your sanitizing is up to you. I'll describe tools and techniques, and you'll choose what seems sensible. Then you'll test to make sure you're getting a lotion that's safe.

What Is Lotion, Anyway?
What It Is and What Goes Into It

Almost any lotion contains a few standard kinds of ingredients. Most of it is plain water or a water-based liquid. Then come fats—oils and butters. Then there's one or more emulsifiers to bring them together. Usually, you'll also have a thickener, an antioxidant, and a preservative. You may also have scent or colorant.

Even the ten-dollar words on commercial lotion bottles fall mostly into one of these categories. They do the same thing as the simpler ingredients we'll work with, and not necessarily any better. There are many other possible additives, but they're optional.

Almost all the ingredients you'll need are available from soapmaking suppliers. A short list of suppliers is included at the end of this book, while a more comprehensive list is on my Soapmaking Page, at www.annelwatson.com.

A word of caution: If you're pregnant, breastfeeding, allergic to nuts, or have other sensitivities, discuss all materials you plan to use in lotionmaking with your health care provider.

When we talk about designing your own lotion, I'll discuss the basic kinds of ingredients in detail and tell you how to balance them. But here's a quick overview to get you started.

Fat

Fats in lotion consist of oils and often butters as well. The origin of the fats may be vegetable, with nut, grain, and seed oils and butters making up the largest part of the handcraft lotionmaker's palette. Or the origin may be animal, as with lanolin or emu oil. Fat can also be replaced entirely with inorganic oil, such as mineral oil—the most common oil in commercial lotion—or a silicone oil such as Dimethicone.

The recipes in this book call for a wide variety of fats—from common ones you'll find in most supermarkets, to exotic specialties that might tempt you in vendor catalogs. You can make good lotion from any of them, and some of the least expensive oils work best.

Water or Other Liquid

Water—or a water-based liquid, such as goat milk or aloe vera gel—is the main ingredient by volume in lotion. Most lotions are 75% to 80% percent water. You can decrease the water content to get a heavier lotion. (Decreasing to about 50% would give you a cream.)

Generally, the water you should use is distilled water. Most water is sanitary, but city tap water is chlorinated and may contain undesirable minerals. And well water is an unknown quantity—it could be fine, or it could be worse than city water.

Emulsifier

Since oil and water normally don't mix, you'll need one or more emulsifiers to combine them. There are many on the market. The two I use in this book are emulsifying wax—its name often shortened to "e-wax"—and conditioning emulsifier, or BTMS. But many others will work if used according to manufacturer's directions.

The consistency of a lotion depends greatly on which emulsifier or emulsifiers you use, and you can adjust that in the recipes in this book. The total amount of emulsifier should remain the same, but you can alter the proportion of emulsifying wax to conditioning emulsifier.

When it comes to consistency, people tend to fall into two camps. Some prefer rich lotion, which you'd make with the emulsifying wax alone. Others prefer a lotion to sink in quickly, and for that you'd use at least some amount of the conditioning emulsifier.

Thickener

The thickener in my recipes is stearic acid, which is inexpensive and widely available. But many others are available. If you prefer another, just use it as recommended by the vendor or manufacturer.

Antioxidant

Antioxidants keeps your fats from going rancid, which is due to a chemical reaction. Don't confuse them with preservatives, which act biologically and do nothing to stop rancidity! The antioxidant I use for my recipes is vitamin E oil.

Preservative

The preservatives I generally use are Germaben II, Germaben IIE (for milk lotions), Germall Plus, and Optiphen. There are many others available as well.

As I've already said, the use of preservative in handmade lotion is controversial. So, I do tell you how to omit them safely for most lotion made for yourself.

Some insurance companies require preservative in any lotion you make for sale. Contrary to what you may often hear, the U.S. Food and Drug Administration does *not* require them. But if a lotion were to spoil or become contaminated with bacteria or mold, the FDA would consider it adulterated, and that would make its sale illegal. Since lotion may go bad without showing any signs of it for some time, selling lotion without preservative is risky.

Some preservatives are more pH sensitive than others. For one of those, you'd have to test your formulation before adding it, to make sure the pH matches the requirements of the preservative. But you don't have to worry about that with the preservatives in my recipes.

A preservative works best within a certain temperature range, and its effectiveness will be reduced if the lotion is too hot when the preservative is added. Find out from your vendor the maximum temperature for your preservative, and make a note of it. Or you may be able to find the information online by searching on the preservative's name.

Generally, it's easier to work with a preservative that has a higher maximum temperature—like Optiphen—because you'll be able to pour the lotion into your bottles while it's still hotter and thinner.

Scent

For scent, you can use any skin-safe fragrance or essential oil. But many people prefer little or no scent, especially in lotion for hands.

If you do use scent, note its *flash point* before you start. You can get this information online or from the vendor. If you add the scent while the lotion temperature is above the flash point, the scent will just evaporate. This doesn't come up with most fragrance oils, but essential oils—especially citrus—may not tolerate nearly the temperature reached by your other ingredients.

Colorant

A colorant can also be added to lotion, though this is not common. If you do want to add it, check with the vendor to make sure the colorant you choose will work for lotion.

In the United States, colorants in lotion for sale are strictly regulated by the FDA. A product is considered adulterated if you don't follow the regulations. Besides needing to be properly listed on the label, a colorant may need to be certified by batch. Even a natural colorant is restricted in some ways. With all these restrictions, you might want to reconsider having a colorant, which adds nothing useful anyway.

Other Additives

Other possibilities include glycerin and other humectants, silk amino acids (silk protein), pH balancers, and many more.

The Two Ways to Sanitize Lotion
And How to Choose Between Them

If handmade lotion is so simple to make, and you wind up with something cheaper and better than commercial products, then why don't more people make it? Why do even soapmakers shy away, when they're used to making cosmetic products from scratch?

Much of it, of course, is from lack of good information about how. But some of it comes down to fears about sanitation—and, if you're selling to others, liability. *What if a germ gets into the lotion? What if it gets moldy? What if it hurts someone?*

I remember when fear of lye stopped many people from making soap. That fear seems to have lessened, as it should have—after all, you can easily test your soap with pH paper to make sure it's safe to use or sell. The good news is, you can test lotion too. There are reliable tests you can have done for you or perform yourself. They can determine whether your formulation and methods are good in general, or they can check specific batches. I discuss those tests later.

It's true that germs and mold are everywhere. But when I looked for instances of a consumer being harmed by lotion, they were hard to find. In fact, the only cases I came across involved either products used near the eyes or contamination in a hospital. You can certainly find people who don't like a particular lotion, or who are allergic to a particular ingredient.

But harm from bacterial or mold contamination of lotion in ordinary use? I couldn't find a thing.

Another reassuring tidbit: In conversation with a representative of the largest insurer of handcraft cosmetics makers, I was told that risk is proportional to the size of your operation. If you make hundreds of bottles of lotion per batch, you'll have some risk. With small batches, insurers regard lotion manufacture as a *low*-risk business.

That told me the problem of sanitation was manageable. But when I started trying to learn *how* to sanitize, I immediately hit a wall of different opinions—many based on fear, and quite a few of them contradictory.

I tried out all the recommendations I could find. What a mess! In the beginning, my kitchen was swimming in bleach water. If you closed your eyes, you might have imagined you were at a public swimming pool. If the place wasn't as sterile as a surgical suite, it wasn't for lack of trying. Then I tried iodophor, and quat sanitizer, and any number of other things.

Making a batch of lotion took most of an exhausting day. Gradually, I started wondering: How much of this did I really need? After all, I'd made my own lotion for years. I'd always worked clean, as if I were preparing food, but I'd never obsessed over sanitation. Yet I'd never had to discard any of it due to spoilage.

That was when I decided to get professional advice. So, I hired a microbiologist as a consultant. Then I made lotion with different sanitizing methods, and had her test them to see which were contaminated.

None of them were. Even the ones for which I'd done no special sanitizing at all.

With those results in hand, I gave a lot of thought to what I'd recommend to my readers. Many, I knew, would make lotion mostly for themselves, and maybe as gifts for friends and family. There seemed little sense in burdening them with procedures they didn't strictly need and that might make the project overwhelming. Others, though, would want to make lotion for sale. For that, they had to meet legal requirements.

In the end, I worked out two parallel approaches—one for making lotion in the simplest way, another for when you need increased sanitation. I call them *Personal Technique* and *Pro Technique*.

Personal Technique is fine for most lotion you make for yourself or those close to you. You'll sanitize your lotion bottles and tops—but other than that, you'll just use clean tools, much the same as if you were preparing a meal.

Pro Technique, with its increased sanitation, could be used for *any* lotionmaking, if you prefer. But you'll *really* need it to make the following:

• Lotion to sell. For commercial lotionmaking, you must follow laws that regulate cosmetics. In practice this means, even if you're making only kinds of lotion that offer little risk, and also using preservative, you must work as if the risk was higher.

• Lotion with perishable ingredients. Many lotions are made with milk or other food ingredients that nourish bacteria and mold. These lotions are more likely than most to spoil.

• Lotion with no preservative. Any lotion is much more likely to spoil if no preservative is used. (Of course, even with increased sanitation, such lotion must be refrigerated and can't be kept long.)

Another case in which you would surely want to use increased sanitation is when making lotion to use on the face, and especially near the eyes. But I won't talk about using Pro Technique for that, because *this book does not recommend making face lotion at all.*

Facial skin is delicate, and may be more prone to breakouts and other reactions than most of your skin. Around your eyes, sanitation is especially crucial. As I said before, almost the only instances I could find of injury from lotion were from when it was used near the eyes.

The lotions in this book, and the procedures for making them, are appropriate for hand and body lotion. I make no claim they're suitable for the face.

I'll go into detail for both Personal Technique and Pro Technique in my instructions on lotionmaking.

What Do I Put It In?
Choosing Your Bottles

The bottles you choose for your lotion should be both practical as containers and aesthetically pleasing. Take some time to choose the bottles and tops that work best for you. And if you're making lotion for sale, be sure to experiment with each combination of bottle, top, and lotion formulation before investing in hundreds of bottles and tops that may prove useless.

Bottles of all types are available from vendors who sell lotion ingredients, and also from container companies. Container companies are likely to offer better prices, but they often require large minimum orders. So, for just a few bottles, stick with your usual vendor, but consider a container company if you're making lotion for sale.

Various plastics are used to make lotion bottles. Different plastics have different temperature tolerances, so check the heat limit of any bottle you're considering.

Bottles come in colored or clear, and also a choice of transparent, translucent, or opaque. In direct sunlight, an opaque bottle will best keep fats from degrading.

Common sizes are two and four fluid ounces. The recipes in this book will fill seven to eight two-ounce bottles.

Two basic shapes are *round* and *oval*—describing the cross section. Among standard bottles, the easiest to sanitize and drain is a round bottle with a rounded shoulder at top—sometimes called a "bullet" shape. Avoid bottles with sharp curves or edges—it's hard to drain them of your sanitizing liquid, and they tend to collect air bubbles when you're filling them with lotion. In general, smoother shapes are easier to work with.

Unlike watery commercial lotions, handcrafted lotions—even light ones—may be too thick to pour or squirt well from standard lotion bottles. You may find you're happier with tottles—also called Malibu tubes—which are designed to stand on their heads. Get a style with a cap large enough for the tottle to stand securely. Tottles, though, do present special problems during filling, which I'll cover in my instructions.

Bottle tops for standard plastic lotion bottles are usually sold separately from the bottles themselves—so don't forget to order! Standard bottles have a number that identifies the size of top they need.

Like bottles, tops are available in many styles and colors. Colors can be chosen to harmonize with your packaging. A style that minimizes finger contact with the lotion will help keep it free of contamination, preserving it longer.

One popular and effective style is the disk top, which pops up on one side to form a spout when the other side is pressed down. A pump top may work well for lotion of light to medium thickness. In fact, a pump may be necessary if the bottle is stiff because of material or shape.

Unlike standard bottles, tottles come with their own tops. The color choice is more limited—usually only white or black.

You may have noticed I've ignored glass bottles. Though you can of course buy these, you generally can't use any tops with them but the simple caps they come with, and these won't keep the lotion away from fingers. Also, unless your lotion is unusually thin, you might not even be able to get it out of the bottle. So, as appealing as glass bottles might be, I can't really recommend them for lotion.

Another thing I don't recommend is reusing lotion bottles and tops. They're almost impossible to get completely clean, and new bottles and tops cost too little to worry about.

What Do I Use to Make It?
Gathering the Equipment You Need

Lotionmaking doesn't involve any hazardous materials or dangerous chemical reactions. So, most of your equipment will be fairly common cooking tools, with a few likely side trips into equipment for restaurants, home brewing, baby feeding, and even car repair. All in all, the things you really need are not expensive.

Below are the items I use or have tried, with a checklist at the end of the chapter. There are probably a hundred possible substitutes for these items. If you think you have something that would work as well or better, you may well be right.

I'll mention which items are needed only for Pro Technique. And as we go on to instructions for lotionmaking, I'll give tips on how to arrange everything efficiently in your work areas.

First off, you need a scale—one that measures accurately at least in grams or tenths of an ounce. A good postal or food scale should do fine. This is one of the few items that have no substitute!

To check temperature, you need a thermometer that includes a range of about 100°–180°F (about 40°–80°C). I prefer a digital thermometer to a candy thermometer, because a candy thermometer is hard to read with lotion all over it. My favorite thermometer is long-stemmed, so it won't fall in the lotion if I let go. But any thermometer with the correct range will do.

For mixing, a stick blender is best. You *could* mix lotion with any number of other tools, including a balloon whip and an electric mixer. But most either are too slow, or they whip in a lot of air. Air isn't fatal to lotion, but the whipped cream texture it creates can make the lotion hard to bottle.

If you prefer to use a countertop blender, you'll need a flat paddle or other beater designed to not whip in air. Be aware that, if the blender's container is plastic instead of glass, lotionmaking may "frost" the inside—though cooling will also be quicker. To prevent running over, the total volume of your lotion ingredients should come to no more than about two-thirds the capacity of the container.

I don't recommend using a food processor. It runs over with very little liquid in it.

As in soapmaking, you need protective clothing while making lotion. This protects your hands and eyes from some ingredients. But unlike in soapmaking, you *mostly* wear it to help keep your product sanitary—in other words, to protect your lotion from *you*.

For Personal Technique, wear freshly laundered clothes to help keep bacteria and mold spores out of your lotion. For Pro Technique, I recommend wearing a clean lab coat or duster. And avoid wearing it at other times—especially outdoors, where there are normally more mold spores to pick up.

It's also a good idea to cover your hair. I use the kind of "hairnet" or "shower cap" made for commercial food workers, and that's what I recommend for Pro Technique. For Personal Technique, you could instead cover it with a scarf, or whatever else you prefer.

Wear gloves. If you make lotion just once in a while, common rubber or disposable gloves will do. If you make lotion professionally, Nitrile or latex powder-free gloves are a worthwhile investment. Whatever kind you use, be sure to get a good fit. If your gloves are too loose, they'll make you clumsy. If too tight, they can tear, causing contamination of the ingredients by your skin.

Goggles should be worn whenever you work directly with a preservative or scent.

To sanitize equipment and bottles, you need a large spray bottle filled with 70% alcohol—commonly called rubbing alcohol or surgical spirit. You also need some kind of drainer—for example, a baby bottle drainer, a cooling rack for bakers, a dish drainer, or even a dishwasher rack. If you're using Pro Technique, my recommendation for this is a bottle tree plus a stainless steel dish drainer and/or cooling racks. (See the picture of a bottle tree opposite this book's title page.) You'll also need a small container for immersing bottle tops—a bowl or plastic tub is fine. And if you prefer not to spray the bottles themselves, you'll need a larger container to immerse them. For countertops, you can spray alcohol or use a general-purpose disinfectant cleanser.

For heating, I recommend a microwave oven for both Personal and Pro techniques, plus a conventional oven for sanitizing in Pro. But you can do it all in a conventional oven instead. You can even heat on a stovetop—but don't heat fats this way without a double boiler. Fats reach their smoke point before you know it, and can even catch fire.

Once you've made your lotion, you have to get it into bottles. There are a number of possible tools for this, and I think I've tried most of them. One I prefer is a large restaurant condiment bottle. Another is a lab burette filler, with a long tube that can reach the bottom of the lotion bottle and fill it up from there.

The screw-on tops found on condiment and similar bottles may or may not be watertight without a little adjustment. Before using one for lotion, fill it with water, turn it upside down over the sink, and see what happens when you squeeze. If water squirts everywhere, lotion will too.

To work around this, you can make a gasket from plastic wrap. With the bottle already full, place a piece of plastic wrap over the top, and let it hang over the edge all around so it also covers the screw-on threads. While holding this piece in place, punch a big hole in the center, so the bottle contents can get through. Then screw on the bottle top, right over the plastic wrap. This trick *should* make the bottle watertight, but again, test it first with water.

Some condiment bottles have very narrow tops, so they can be a challenge to fill. This is especially true when you're using a preservative needing a lower temperature and your lotion has cooled enough to thicken. One of my best discoveries has been to make this easier with a large vented funnel. Tiny grooves on the outside, where the funnel contacts the bottle's neck, allow air *out* of the bottle so lotion can keep flowing *in*. My funnel came from an automotive store, but labs use them, too. A smaller vented funnel, sold as a kitchen item, can be used if you prefer to fill lotion bottles directly, instead of with a filling tool.

Other possibilities for filling tools include plastic bags and cake decorating bags. But those are floppy and awkward, taking both hands to use them—which leaves you one hand short for holding the bottle you're filling. You can get around this by using something else to hold your bottles steady. I've done fairly well with a baby bottle drying rack, setting bottles upright between prongs.

You'll also need the following common equipment and supplies, most of which you may already have in your kitchen:

• Weighing containers. I use one for oil phase ingredients together, one for water phase ingredients together, and one for each cool down phase ingredient—generally, preservative and scent. Ordinary kitchen bowls, mason jars, measuring pitchers, and other common containers work well. I avoid silicone containers because they can absorb odors. Although only tiny amounts of preservative and scent are used, these containers should still each hold at least a cup (about a quarter liter).

• Heating containers—one for oil phase ingredients together, and one for water phase ingredients together. I prefer mason jars, but Pyrex pitchers are fine, too. In any case, the containers should be microwave safe, and for Pro Technique, also ovenproof. For the recipes in this book, pint (half-liter) containers work well most of the time. The exception is when you're using Pro Technique and the water phase ingredients include one like milk that might run over when heated. In that case, put those ingredients in a larger container—say, one that holds a quart (about a liter)—or else split them between two smaller ones. For mason jars with Pro Technique, you should also have metal lids and screw bands.

• Mixing container. This container should hold about a quart (about a liter)—more than enough for the recipes in this book. For use with a stick blender, it should be cylindrical, and the diameter should be no more than about 5½ inches (about 14 centimeters). This is because, if the lotion is spread out and too shallow, you'll have trouble keeping the head of your stick blender covered, and you'll wind up whipping air into the mixture. Also, for quicker cooling, you might prefer a container that does not retain heat, such as one made of plastic or thin metal.

A number of kinds of container meet these requirements. A tall plastic pitcher will work just fine. Or you may prefer a pitcher of stainless steel—for example, a milk frothing pitcher for making espresso.

A metal pot can work too. Best would be one that's tall but relatively small in diameter—like an asparagus pot. Just be aware that high-quality, gourmet cookware of this kind comes with a slight disadvantage: The heat-retaining core on its bottom will slow down cooling.

• Plastic pipettes, baby medicine droppers, large eyedroppers, or plastic straws. When weighing, any of these are good for adding or subtracting small amounts of liquid. Here's how to use a straw for this: Set it upright in the liquid, press your forefinger over the opening at the top to make an airtight seal, and lift out the straw with your finger in place. To release a few drops, ease the pressure on your finger to let in a little air, then quickly reseal. To release it all, just lift off your finger.

• A few spoons or scoops. Avoid wooden implements—it's hard to keep them clean enough.

• Long-handled spoon.

• One to three rubber or silicone spatulas. Avoid ones with wooden handles.

• One or two canning funnels (optional). These are handy if any of your containers are jars rather than pitchers.

• Pot holders. Flexible knitted oven gloves work best.

• Trivet or folded towel (optional). For hot containers to sit on.

• Dishpan or soup pot (optional). With this, you can speed cooling by giving your mixing container a cold water bath.

• Plastic wrap. For covering containers.

• Cheesecloth. For covering lotion bottles.

• Distilled water. Besides any that's called for in the recipe, you'll need this to compensate for evaporation during heating.

• Tray (optional). For lotion bottles being filled.

• Rubber bands (optional). To band tottles together for stability while filling.

• Filling syringe (optional). To inject more lotion into a tottle after capping, if necessary.

• Roasting pan or other shallow pan (for Pro Technique only). Something you can use in the oven. A brownie pan and a lasagna pan are other possibilities.

• Aluminum foil or silicone lids (for jars without tight lids, in Pro Technique only).

• Jar opener (for mason jars with Pro Technique only).

• Kitchen timer (optional, for Pro Technique only).

Equipment Checklist

Scale

Thermometer, preferably digital long-stem

Stick blender (preferred) or other mixer

Hair covering; for Pro Technique, restaurant "hairnet" or
"shower cap"

Gloves, rubber or disposable; for Pro Technique, Nitrile or
latex powder-free

Goggles

70% alcohol

Spray bottle (for alcohol)

Drainer—baby bottle, dish, cooling rack, dishwasher rack, or
other; for Pro Technique, bottle tree plus stainless steel
dish drainer and/or cooling racks

Small container for alcohol bath (for tops)

Large container for alcohol bath (optional, for bottles)

Disinfectant cleanser (optional)

Microwave oven (preferred), conventional oven, or double
boiler

Condiment bottle, lab burette filler, or other filling tool

Vented funnel, large (optional, for condiment bottle)

Weighing containers, four or more

Heating containers, two, one-pint (half-liter), microwave-
safe; for Pro Technique, also ovenproof, with additional
container, one-quart (liter) or one-pint (half-liter)

Mixing container

Pipettes, droppers, or plastic drinking straws (optional)

Spoons or scoops
Long-handled spoon
Spatulas, one to three
Canning funnels, one or two (optional, for jars)
Pot holders
Trivet or folded towel (optional)
Dishpan or soup pot (optional, for cold water bath)
Plastic wrap
Cheesecloth
Distilled water
Tray (optional)
Rubber bands (optional, for tottles)
Filling syringe (optional, for tottles)

For Pro Technique only:

Lab coat or duster
Conventional oven (in addition to microwave)
Metal lids and screw bands (for mason jars)
Roasting pan or other shallow oven pan
Aluminum foil or silicone lids (for heating containers without tight lids)
Jar opener (for mason jars)
Kitchen timer (optional)

Anne's Almond Lotion

Here's a recipe that's ideal for your first lotion. It's a medium to light lotion with a silky feel. Almond oil gives you that—which is why it's one of my favorite ingredients. But if you're allergic to nuts, you can substitute sunflower or meadowfoam oil for the almond.

Use this formulation as you go through the steps in the next chapter. It's handy to copy the recipe so you don't have to flip pages back and forth.

Oil Phase

> 54 grams (1.9 ounces) almond oil
> 13 grams (.5 ounce) stearic acid
> 23 grams (.8 ounce) emulsifying wax
> 5 grams (.2 ounce) vitamin E oil

Water Phase

> 354 grams (12.5 ounces) distilled water

Cool Down Phase

> 5 grams (.2 ounce) Germaben II or Optiphen
> Up to 6 grams (.2 ounce) scent (optional)

**Before using this recipe, read the following pages
thoroughly to understand the method!**

Step-by-Step Lotionmaking
From Prep to Cleanup and Beyond

There are just a few basic steps to making lotion, and here they are:

1. Weigh the ingredients.
2. Heat the ingredients.
3. Mix the ingredients.

Simple, right? Now let's look at these procedures in detail, adding in preliminaries and follow-up.

Unless marked, the instructions apply to both Personal and Pro techniques. Where they differ, you'll see side-by-side instructions with different shading, like so:

Personal Technique	**Pro Technique**
Instructions go here!	Instructions go here!

Sanitizing Your Workspace

When you make lotion, everything has to be clean or sanitized, and that starts with working in a clean, sanitary environment. Work in a room that's not subject to mold. The room should be warm and normally well ventilated—though for the time you're sanitizing and making lotion, you should keep windows closed.

Keep sources of bacteria, molds, and yeasts out of the area or securely closed up. Some foods and beverages contain them—peanuts, bread dough, yogurt, and wine, for example. Avoid eating and drinking while making lotion. And don't make lotion when you're sick.

Set out a trash container in the open—a paper grocery bag is perfect. This lets you avoid touching cabinet doors or trash-can lids while you work. And you *will* generate a small amount of trash, which you'd be wise to dispose of immediately, rather than letting it clutter your work area.

Clean your countertops thoroughly before you start. I use a bleach-based disinfectant cleanser for this. Or you can spray the counters with 70% alcohol. If your countertops are made of something that shouldn't be treated like that—or if it's just more convenient—you can cover them with sheet vinyl or plastic shelf liner and sanitize the covering.

Sanitizing Equipment and Supplies

For anything other than countertops, 70% alcohol is the safest and most effective sanitizer. Avoid sanitizers like chlorine bleach, quaternary sanitizer, iodophor sanitizer, and medical sanitizers such as chlorhexidine. Even when properly diluted, these products can leave odors, or residues that cause skin reactions.

Here's what you'll need for sanitizing with alcohol:

- Spray bottle
- Small container (for soaking bottle tops)

- Large container (optional, for soaking bottles)
- Rubber gloves (optional)

You'll also need one or more drainers:

Personal Technique	Pro Technique
• Baby bottle drainer, cooling rack, dish drainer, dishwasher rack, or other drainer	• Bottle tree • Stainless steel dish drainer and/or cooling racks

Alcohol is not an especially dangerous material, but it can be rough on your hands. So, you might want to wear rubber gloves while sanitizing. Goggles and other protective wear are not needed for this.

Bottles and Tops

Assuming you're using new bottles and tops, they're not likely to need washing before you sanitize them. They should already be clean, unless they've been contaminated since coming out of their packaging. That's something you should be able to judge by sight.

In fact, if your bottles and tops come in sealed plastic packages, they're almost certainly sterile as well. But sanitizing is quick and easy, so I still advise it as a safety measure—and of course, you would never omit it for Pro Technique.

Before sanitizing your bottles, sanitize the drainer or drainers you'll set them on by spraying thoroughly with alcohol. Then follow this procedure:

1. Spray the interior of each bottle with alcohol. Make sure the alcohol covers the inner surface completely.

2. Drain the alcohol.

3. Repeat the alcohol spray.

4. Drain again, this time being careful to shake any pooled alcohol out of the bottle shoulder.

5. Set the bottle upside down on the drainer. Allow the alcohol to evaporate until you can no longer smell it.

Here's an alternate method:

1. Submerge each bottle in an alcohol bath in a large container. Make sure to eliminate any air bubbles from inside the bottle. While it's soaking, you can cover the container with a lid or plastic wrap to minimize fumes.

2. Remove the bottle after about a minute and drain it, being careful to shake any pooled alcohol out of the shoulder.

3. Set the bottle upside down on the drainer. Allow the alcohol to evaporate until you can no longer smell it.

Next is sanitizing your bottle tops (including any pumps):

1. Dunk each piece in an alcohol bath in a small container.

2. Remove it after about a minute and shake off excess alcohol.

3. Set it on the drainer. Allow the alcohol to evaporate until you can no longer smell it.

It's much better to sanitize your bottles and tops the night before you make lotion. That way, the alcohol has plenty of time to evaporate completely.

If that's not convenient, you might be able to cut the evaporation time down to a couple of hours—at least on a warm, dry day. First spray the bottles as I've described and let them drain upside down for one hour; then turn them upright and leave them for another hour to let the alcohol evaporate. But whether this works that quickly depends on temperature and humidity, so I can't guarantee it.

You can also sanitize a large batch of bottles and tops far ahead of time, then seal them in a plastic bag until you're ready to use them. I've done this and later had the bottles tested, and they were still sanitary.

Tools and Containers

In general, cleaning comes before sanitizing. Wash all tools and containers thoroughly by hand with hot water and a good dishwashing soap, or in the dishwasher. Allow to air dry.

That's really all you need to do to them for Personal Technique. For Pro Technique, go on to sanitize all tools and containers that will touch lotion ingredients or even another piece of equipment. Here's the method:

Personal Technique	Pro Technique
Don't do a thing!	1. Sanitize your drainer or drainers by spraying thoroughly with alcohol. 2. Spray each tool or container with alcohol until it's dripping. 3. Turn upside down on drainer. Allow the alcohol to evaporate until you can no longer smell it.

If you sanitize your equipment very long before you plan to use it, you can protect it with a covering of plastic wrap.

Dressing for Lotionmaking

After sanitizing, you want to minimize the chances of contaminating anything yourself, as well as to protect yourself from ingredients that might harm you. For Pro Technique, you should have an entire special outfit that you use only when making lotion. On the other hand, you don't normally need to go that far just to make a few bottles for yourself.

Here's what you should wear for lotionmaking:

Personal Technique	Pro Technique
• Freshly washed clothes • Hair covering • Rubber or disposable gloves • Goggles	• Clean lab coat or duster • Restaurant "hairnet" or "shower cap" • Nitrile or latex powder-free gloves • Goggles

Goggles are needed only while weighing and mixing ingredients like preservative and scent. You don't need them at other times. I'll tell you when to put them on.

You don't need a surgical mask, as is sometimes recommended to protect lotion from viruses. Common viruses won't survive in lotion, and wouldn't likely be transmitted if they did.

While dressed for lotionmaking, avoid touching anything that hasn't been sanitized or at least cleaned. That includes children, plants, and pets! If you do touch something risky, change your gloves, or spray alcohol on them and wait about thirty seconds for it to work. This is especially important for Pro Technique.

Preparing the Work Areas

Now that everything's sanitized or cleaned and you're properly dressed, you need to set up three work areas for lotionmaking: a weighing area, a heating and mixing area, and a bottling area.

Weighing Area

Here's what you'll put in your weighing area:

- All recipe ingredients
- Scale
- Weighing containers, four or more
- Spoons or scoops
- Pipettes, droppers, or plastic drinking straws (optional)
- Spatula
- Canning funnel (optional)
- Plastic wrap
- Distilled water (if not already a recipe ingredient)

You'll also need to put your heating containers in this area:

The Weighing Area

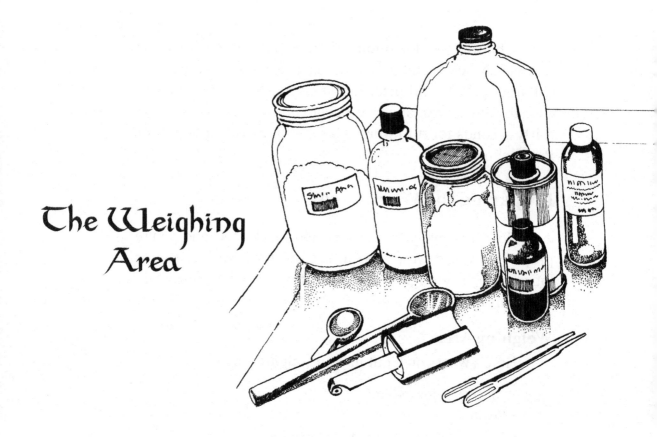

Personal Technique	**Pro Technique**
• Heating containers, two, one-pint (half-liter), microwave-safe	• Heating containers, two, one-pint (half-liter), microwave-safe and ovenproof

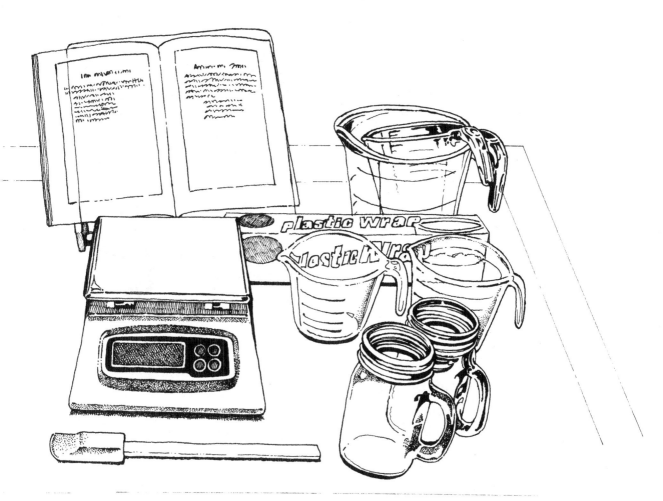

Though you won't have to worry about this for our starter recipe, or for Personal Technique in general, some water phase ingredients like milk could run over if heated for a prolonged period. So, if you're using Pro Technique with such an ingredient, substitute a larger heating container for one of the smaller ones, or else have an additional small one so you can split the water phase ingredients between two.

If you have ingredients in containers you've never opened, open them before you start. It's frustrating to stop to unseal bottles when you're trying to concentrate on weighing things correctly.

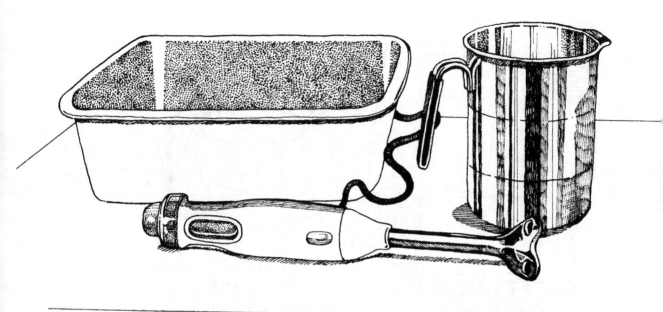

Heating and Mixing Area

The heating and mixing area should be close to the microwave, and also to the conventional oven, if you're using Pro Technique. Here's what goes there:

- Thermometer
- Pot holders
- Trivet or folded towel (optional)
- Mixing container
- Canning funnel (optional)
- Stick blender (or other mixer)
- Long-handled spoon
- Dishpan or soup pot with cold water (optional)
- Spatula

For Pro Technique, add:

The Heating and Mixing Area

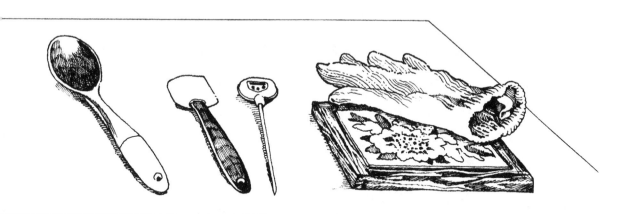

Personal Technique	Pro Technique
Nothing more!	• Roasting pan or other shallow oven pan • Metal lids and screw bands (for mason jars) • Aluminum foil or silicone lids (for heating containers without tight lids) • Kitchen timer (optional) • Jar opener (for mason jars)

For Pro Technique, also go ahead and set up a hot water bath, like so:

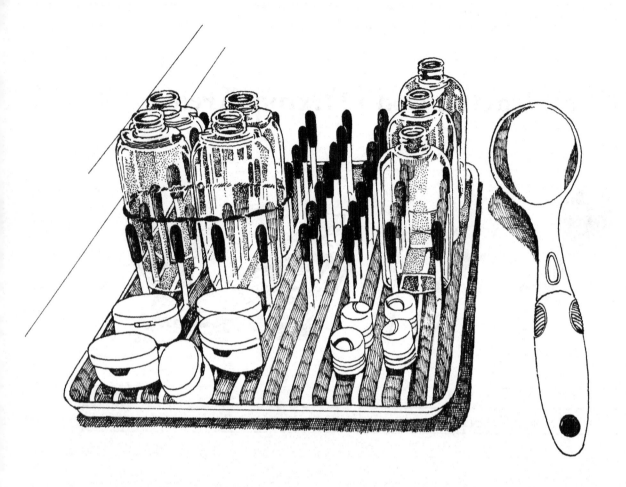

Personal Technique	Pro Technique
Don't do a thing!	1. Place the roasting pan in your conventional oven.
	2. Fill the pan with water to a depth of about an inch (about 2 cm).
	3. Preheat to about 180°F (about 80°C).

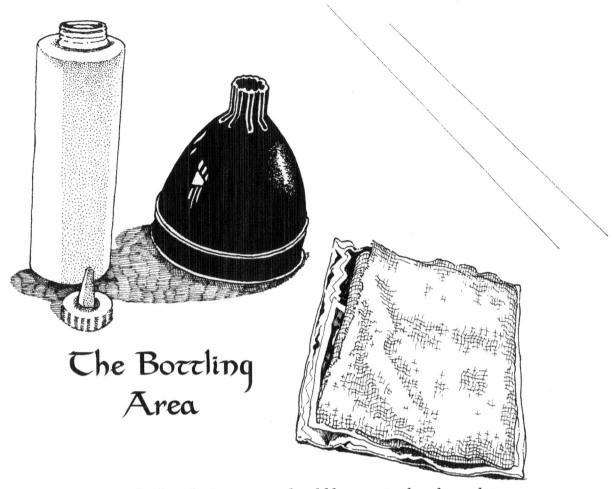

The Bottling Area

For both techniques, you should keep notes handy on the maximum temperature of your preservative and the flash point of your scent, to tell you how much you need to let the lotion cool before adding these ingredients.

Bottling Area

The bottling area should be close to the heating and mixing area, but avoid having things crowded. If you have a messy, confused work area, it's easy to make mistakes.

Here's what goes in the bottling area:

- Lotion bottles and tops
- Condiment bottle (or other filling tool)
- Vented funnel, large (optional, for condiment bottle)
- Spatula
- Tray or baby bottle drainer (optional)
- Rubber bands (optional, for tottles)
- Cheesecloth
- Filling syringe (optional, for tottles)

Weighing the Ingredients

Though all my recipes include weight in both grams and ounces, I recommend weighing in grams—even if you're not used to it. Grams are just more accurate, since there are about 28 of them to the ounce.

It's important not to lose track of what you're doing. Many lotionmaking ingredients look alike, so you need a system of organization to make sure you handle them correctly. For myself, I put all ingredients into a box as I take them off the shelves, then set the box beside my scale. After weighing and adding each ingredient, I set down its container *outside the box*. This simple system keeps me from missing anything.

Even with such a system, check your recipe often and pay close attention as you work. For example, when adding emulsifying wax, I may start by noting I need 26 grams. I pick up the jar of e-wax, check the label, and recheck the recipe to make sure I haven't misread the quantity. I weigh the 26 grams of e-wax, check the label again to make sure the jar in my hand really is e-wax, and put the jar down. I check the scale again to make sure it reads 26 grams, and refer to the recipe one more time to make sure that 26 grams of e-wax is really *really* what I want. Only then do I add it to the other ingredients.

Yes, it's repetitious and sounds ridiculous—until you've made a few bad mistakes and ruined a few batches. (And, take my word for it, everyone does that—or almost does it—sooner or later.) Once this kind of checking becomes a habit, it takes only a few seconds, and it virtually eliminates errors.

Not quite, though. You need to do one more thing: Learn to know when something *looks* wrong.

Here's one example. As I weighed and added ingredients for one of my test lotions, I could see that the oil phase had far too little oil in it—there just wasn't enough in the jar. Probably I'd tared my scale *before* I put the container on it. Or maybe I'd read the *ounce* amount in the recipe as *grams*. Whatever it was, I could tell I'd made a bad mistake. So, I reweighed my ingredients, corrected my error, and went on to make a fine batch of lotion.

You'll start by weighing the oil phase ingredients and adding them to each other. Then you'll do the same for the water phase ingredients. Finally, you'll weigh the cool down phase ingredients—primarily preservative and scent—to add later.

Here are the steps for each of these.

Oil Phase Ingredients

1. Set one of your weighing containers on the scale. Turn the scale on or tare it, so it reads zero.

2. Weigh out the needed amount of your first oil phase ingredient.

3. Pour the ingredient into one of your heating containers. If necessary, scrape the inside of the weighing container with a

spatula. Because my heating containers are mason jars, I use a canning funnel to add ingredients.

4. Using the same weighing and heating containers, repeat the steps above for all other oil phase ingredients.

5. Cover the heating container tightly with plastic wrap and move it to your heating and mixing area.

Here's a tip that makes weighing solid ingredients much easier—if your scale registers negative numbers. Suppose I need 12 grams of emulsifying wax. I put my open jar of e-wax on the scale and tare it. I then scoop out e-wax, adding it directly to my heating container, until the scale reads -12 grams. I didn't need a measuring container at all!

One more tip: Suppose your lotion has a particularly sticky ingredient, like shea butter. Weigh that first, but in the *heating* container, and just leave it in there. That way, you won't have to transfer it from the weighing container.

Water Phase Ingredients

1. Set your other weighing container on the scale and tare.

2. Weigh out the needed amount of your first water phase ingredient.

3. Pour the ingredient into your other heating container. Use a spatula if necessary, and a canning funnel if you like.

4. With the same weighing and heating containers, repeat the steps above for any other water phase ingredients.

5. When all water phase ingredients have been measured out and added to the heating container, tare the scale with *nothing* on it.

6. Weigh the heating container *with* its contents and write down the weight. (You'll need this later to tell how much has evaporated during heating.)

7. Cover the heating container tightly with plastic wrap and move it to your heating and mixing area.

As in our starter recipe, often the formulation has only one water phase ingredient—typically, distilled water. In that case, you can weigh it directly in the heating container. Just remember, after measuring the ingredient *without* the weight of the container, you must then also measure their *combined* weight.

Cool Down Phase Ingredients

1. Put on your goggles.

2. Set a weighing container on the scale and tare it.

3. Weigh out the needed amount of your first cool down phase ingredient.

4. Cover the weighing container with plastic wrap and move it to your heating and mixing area.

5. With *different* weighing containers, repeat the steps above for any other cool down phase ingredients.

6. Take off your goggles.

Heating the Ingredients

The heating part of the procedure brings your ingredients to a good working temperature for mixing and bottling.

With Pro Technique, it also sanitizes your ingredients. Though your preservative might do that adequately by itself, the prolonged heating described here is an extra measure of safety. Of course, it becomes more important if you're using perishable ingredients like milk or other food items—and it's essential if you're not using preservative.

Personal Technique	Pro Technique
1. Put the oil phase heating container into the microwave with the plastic wrap still on. Heat in thirty-second bursts until most of the solid ingredients are melted. This will probably take a total time between a minute and 90 seconds, depending on your microwave.	1. If you haven't already done it, set up a hot water bath. Place your roasting pan in your conventional oven, fill the pan with water to a depth of about one inch (about two centimeters), and preheat to about 180°F (about 80°C). The *water* must reach that temperature, not just the oven!
2. Remove the container from the microwave, take off the plastic wrap, stir, then let sit a few seconds. In most cases, all remaining solids will then melt. If not, replace the plastic wrap and return the container to the microwave for more heating, then stir again. But don't overheat! If you take any fat to its smoke point, it's no longer usable.	2. Put the oil phase heating container into the microwave with the plastic wrap still on. Heat in thirty-second bursts until most of the solid ingredients are melted. This will probably take a total time between a minute and 90 seconds, depending on your microwave.
3. Put the water phase heating container into the microwave with the plastic wrap still on and heat it. Though this temperature is not critical, aim for very warm but not too hot to hold. This might take a minute or two, depending on your microwave.	3. Remove the container from the microwave, take off the plastic wrap, stir, then check the temperature. You want it about 180°F (about 80°C). As needed, replace the plastic wrap and return the container to the microwave for more heating until you reach that temperature. But don't overheat! If you

Personal Technique	Pro Technique

4. Take this container back to the weighing area and weigh it with its contents to see how much water has evaporated. Add distilled water as needed to bring the weight back to your original measurement. (It doesn't matter whether distilled water was the original ingredient.) Return the container to the heating and mixing area.

take any fat to its smoke point, it's no longer usable.

4. Replace the plastic wrap with the metal jar lid, tightly-fitted aluminum foil, or silicone lid and place the container into the pre-heated water bath in the oven.

5. Put the water phase heating container into the microwave with the plastic wrap still on and heat it to about 180°F (about 80°C). Do not let it boil. Replace the plastic wrap with the metal jar lid, tightly-fitted aluminum foil, or silicone lid and place the container into the preheated water bath in the oven.

6. Leave the containers in the oven for twenty minutes. (I recommend using a timer.)

7. Turn off the oven and move the containers carefully to a trivet or cooling rack. Remove the lids or aluminum foil. (If you're using mason jar lids, you might need a jar opener for that, as the jars sometimes seal in the oven.)

Personal Technique	Pro Technique
	8. Take the water phase container back to the weighing area and weigh it with its contents to see how much water has evaporated. Add distilled water as needed to bring the weight back to your original measurement. (It doesn't matter whether distilled water was the original ingredient. It also doesn't matter if this small amount didn't go through the hot water bath.) Return the container to the heating and mixing area.

Mixing the Ingredients

1. Pour the oil phase ingredients into your mixing container.

2. Pour the water phase ingredients into the oil phase heating container—no, not yet into the mixing container! The hot liquid will pick up any residue from the oil phase ingredients (and probably turn white). This will get all your precious fat into the lotion, and will also make the jar much easier to wash. With a jar, you might want to use a canning funnel.

3. Pour the water phase ingredients from the oil phase heating container into the mixing container.

4. Mix with the stick blender for about 15 seconds. Try not to let the head of the stick blender break the surface of the

liquid. The point here is to avoid beating too much air into the lotion. Also, don't blend too long, or the lotion will get foamy.

5. Hand stir for a minute or two with your long-handled spoon to get rid of air bubbles. The mixture should still be very thin.

6. If necessary, let the mixture cool enough to reach the prescribed temperature range of your preservative and scent. For Germaben II, for instance, the recommended maximum temperature is 140°F (60°C). For Optiphen, it's 176°F (80°C)—high enough that it might not require you to cool at all. For scent, you must cool the lotion below the flash point of the fragrance or essential oil before adding.

Cooling to the proper range can take a few minutes, or it can take much longer, depending on the container, the quantity of lotion, and how much heat you need to lose. Check temperature often, and don't let the lotion cool much more than your preservative and scent require. If it gets too cool, it will be hard to bottle, and the emulsion may break down if you reheat.

If you like, speed up this process by putting your mixing container into a dishpan of cold water. Stir as it's cooling. This cold water bath will cool the lotion quickly, so don't take your eye off it or your thermometer out of it. Again, don't cool the lotion more than you have to. Also, don't let go of the mixing container even for a second, since it may overturn as it floats.

7. Put on your goggles.

8. As soon as the lotion is cool enough, pour a little into one of your weighing containers that holds a cool down phase ingredient (such as a preservative or scent). Stick blend for about 15 seconds to mix thoroughly. Pour back into the mixing container, using a spatula to get the last of it. Stir well with your long-handled spoon.

9. Repeat as needed for each cool down phase ingredient.
10. Take off your goggles.
11. Move the lotion to the bottling area.

Bottling the Lotion

These instructions assume you're using a condiment bottle as your filling tool, but of course, you can use something different. In fact, using a funnel, you can even fill your bottles directly from your mixing container—though it's much more awkward.

If you're working with a large amount of lotion—more than my recipes make—you might divide the lotion before bottling and keep part of it warm, to keep it from congealing before you get to it.

1. Using your large vented funnel, pour the lotion into the condiment bottle. Use a spatula to get the last of it from the mixing container. Screw the cap on the condiment bottle, making sure it's tight.

2. Fill your individual lotion bottles from the condiment bottle. To avoid foaming, direct the stream of lotion toward the side of the bottle, not straight downward. If your lotion is more runny, you can get more control by tilting the lotion bottle while the nozzle of the condiment bottle is inside. You may want to work with your lotion bottles on a tray or baby bottle drainer to reduce mess.

Tottles require slightly different handling than standard bottles do. For one thing, they're rounded on top—on the part that on a regular bottle would be the base. So, when they're upside down for filling, it's hard to get them to stay upright. To make them less tippy, you can rubber-band several of them together.

Also, a tottle must be filled completely—including the neck—or you'll wind up with a visible air bubble on top. This doesn't matter if you're making lotion for yourself, but it's probably not something you want if you're selling lotion or giving it to someone.

Whichever kind of bottle you have, avoid introducing air pockets into it—and especially avoid blocking the neck with lotion before the bottle is full. If you do get a pocket, cap the lotion bottle temporarily and tap the base of it against your work surface. Or, with a tottle, use plastic wrap instead to cover the opening while you tap, since a cap cannot be removed once in place.

4. With the bottles still uncapped, cover them loosely with cheesecloth and let them cool completely. (Leaving off the cap avoids water condensing under it.) Depending on the size of bottle and how much space you leave around them, cooling can take up to several hours.

5. With the lotion at room temperature, cap the bottles.

For perfect filling, a tottle should be topped off just before it's capped. Cover the opening with plastic wrap and tap the other end against your work surface a few times to make sure the lotion is settled. Then add enough lotion to fill to the top of the neck.

If somehow your tottle develops an air bubble *after* capping, you can use a filling syringe to force a little more lotion into it.

Cleanup

If you use an automatic dishwasher, first hand wash your utensils and containers. If you don't, your entire load of dishes will come out with an oily film.

If you're washing *only* by hand, soap twice to remove the residue.

After Lotionmaking

Keep the bottles somewhere with moderate to cool temperature, out of direct sunlight. If the lotion is preservative-free, keep it refrigerated and discard after a week to ten days.

It's very tempting to try your lotion right away, but I suggest you wait. Though your lotion will thicken at least a bit as it cools, it may not completely set and stop being liquid for eight to twelve hours, or even longer. Don't worry, though. As long as it's completely emulsified, with no layering, it's on track.

Beyond that, I find that a lotion and the feel of it changes over a period of a week or so after it's made—more in the beginning. Of course, if you didn't use a preservative, you won't be able to wait so long!

If you're not satisfied with a lotion even after it's had time to settle down, see the chapter on troubleshooting for tips on how to modify your recipe.

Handcrafted lotions in general are thicker than commercial lotions—I think you'll like the difference. Within their range, though, you may find you prefer different "weights" in different seasons. A heavier lotion may protect your skin from chapping in severe winter weather but feel too heavy and dense in warmer, drier weather.

Testing Your Lotion
Making Sure It's Safe

Contamination of lotion is not as likely as you might imagine, but it can happen if your sanitizing doesn't kill enough of the bacteria and molds in your environment, or if your formulation doesn't allow for careless use. So, even if you're not selling your lotion, I still recommend testing, if only for your peace of mind.

If you *are* selling your lotion, you'll need to test more rigorously. Testing may or may not be required by government agencies or by insurers—in the United States, for instance, it is not technically required by the Food and Drug Administration. But it is still the only way to be sure your lotion is legal to sell and to avoid liability. Beyond that, you have a duty to your customers to guarantee the safety of your product.

There are two kinds of safety tests for bacteria and mold. The first kind counts living microorganisms that remain and multiply after lotionmaking. The *aerobic plate count* (for bacteria) and the *fungal/yeast count* (for molds) will tell you whether your methods have given you lotion that's sufficiently sanitary. If you're selling lotion, you should apply these tests to each and every batch. If making lotion for family or friends, apply them when you're starting out, and after that as often as necessary to be confident of your methods.

You can have these done professionally, and they're not expensive. Or you can do them yourself, with a home testing kit. In fact, once you grasp the basics, you can buy the ingredients individually from science supply vendors for some savings.

What if your lotion doesn't pass? Then add some or all of the Pro Technique to your procedure—even if you're not making lotion that would otherwise require it. It's unlikely you'll need to do that, but you can't know for sure unless you test.

The second kind of test is called a *challenge test,* because your lotion is "challenged" by intentionally introducing bacteria and molds. The samples are tested and retested over a period of four weeks. For your lotion to pass, the bacteria and molds must *decrease,* returning to a safe level.

This kind of testing is needed only if you're selling lotion. It's a test more of your formulation and its preservative than of your methods, so for each formulation, it's done only once. That's lucky, because this one *must* be done by a professional, and it's not cheap.

Because of the expense, you might want to first run an informal version yourself. This is called a *common usage test,* and it at least gives you an idea what results to expect from the challenge test.

To run this, first test a sample of your lotion for existing bacteria and molds, and then "challenge" it—leave the lotion exposed to open air, touch it with dirty fingers, and such. Test again in two weeks to see whether bacteria and molds have returned to acceptable levels, as your testing kit defines.

For professional testing, there's a brief list of U.S. labs at the back of this book. You can also search online for "cosmetic testing lab," or contact your regional soapmaking guild.

Another useful test is a pH test, if you suspect a lotion has gone bad. The usual pH range for lotion is between 5 and 7, which is slightly acidic. A lotion with active bacterial contamination may have a very high or low pH—above 8 or below 4. This is a quick way to tell whether contamination is likely.

More Recipes!
Different Lotions You Can Try

Now you're ready to try a variety of basic lotions that are easy to make. These all work with the same setup and instructions already given.

Recipes are for small, personal-size batches—about one pound (about half a kilogram) of lotion. For larger batches, simply increase the measurements proportionally—for instance, for a two-pound batch, you'd just double everything.

The descriptions include my opinions about how the lotions feel, and the opinions of my testers. But these are mostly *not* the kinds of statements you could put on a commercial label, so I don't recommend quoting them on one! (If you're selling lotion, see the section on commercial labeling.)

All ounce measurements are rounded to the nearest tenth. But even with tenths of ounces, grams are more exact, and that's what I've used when designing the recipes. If you're not used to working in grams, this would be a good chance to try it.

Several lotions call for coconut oil. Unless the recipe says otherwise, this is plain coconut oil—sometimes called "76-degree" coconut oil, after its Fahrenheit melting point. Though there are other kinds, they'll be clearly identified by the vendor. So, any oil you find that just says "Coconut Oil" should be safe to use.

Another ingredient that can cause confusion is aloe vera gel. This is actually a liquid, and may be called aloe vera liquid by the soapmaking and lotion suppliers that carry it. Don't confuse it with the burn medication that's likewise known as aloe vera gel and really *is* one. Also, don't confuse it with aloe vera juice, a health food drink. Also be aware that there's an aloe vera oil or extract oil that's something else entirely.

Silk amino acids may also be called silk protein. Shea oil may be called shea olein.

Another common name for conditioning emulsifier is BTMS. Emulsifying wax may also be called e-wax.

For preservative, most recipes list Germaben II and Optiphen as two choices. The measurement of 5 grams (.2 ounce) is based on the manufacturer's recommendation for Germaben II and *minimum* recommendation for Optiphen—so, if you feel the need, you can increase the amount of Optiphen up to the maximum, which would be 7 grams (.25 ounce). You can use any other preservative instead, as long as you follow the manufacturer's directions. Or you can omit preservative, if you follow the directions given earlier for Pro Technique.

The amounts for scent are a maximum. If you prefer subtle scent, you'll probably want to use less. Or you can just leave it out.

Anne's Walnut Lotion

This lotion feels light and silky, but it's also rich and has a long-lasting effect. For my own skin and climate, it's perfect. Out of all the lotions I've designed or tested, this is the one I make for myself.

Oil Phase

 60 grams (2.1 ounces) walnut oil
 8 grams (.3 ounce) stearic acid
 14 grams (.5 ounce) conditioning emulsifier
 6 grams (.2 ounce) vitamin E oil

Water Phase

 361 grams (12.7 ounces) distilled water

Cool Down Phase

 5 grams (.2 ounce) Germaben II or Optiphen
 Up to 6 grams (.2 ounce) scent (optional)

Shea Lotion

This lotion is especially good for cold, dry weather.

Oil Phase

    65 grams (2.3 ounces) shea oil
    7 grams (.2 ounce) shea butter
    20 grams (.7 ounce) emulsifying wax
    3 grams (.1 ounce) conditioning emulsifier
    5 grams (.2 ounce) vitamin E oil

Water Phase

    335 grams (11.8 ounces) distilled water
    22 grams (.8 ounce) silk amino acids

Cool Down Phase

    5 grams (.2 ounce) Germaben II or Optiphen
    Up to 6 grams (.2 ounce) scent (optional)

California Lotion

A well-balanced lotion—light, but somehow creamy, too. Grapes and avocado—what could be more California?

Oil Phase

    37 grams (1.3 ounces) grapeseed oil
    6 grams (.2 ounce) avocado oil
    6 grams (.2 ounce) avocado butter
    11 grams (.4 ounce) stearic acid
    23 grams (.8 ounce) emulsifying wax
    5 grams (.2 ounce) vitamin E oil

Water Phase

    360 grams (12.7 ounces) distilled water

Cool Down Phase

    5 grams (.2 ounce) Germaben II or Optiphen
    Up to 6 grams (.2 ounce) scent (optional)

Sunflower and Avocado Lotion

A favorite of a friend in Arizona. Sunflower oil and avocado butter make an especially emollient mixture.

Oil Phase

> 37 grams (1.3 ounces) sunflower oil
> 14 grams (.5 ounce) avocado butter
> 9 grams (.3 ounce) stearic acid
> 23 grams (.8 ounce) emulsifying wax
> 6 grams (.2 ounce) vitamin E oil

Water Phase

> 360 grams (12.7 ounces) distilled water

Cool Down Phase

> 5 grams (.2 ounce) Germaben II or Optiphen
> Up to 6 grams (.2 ounce) scent (optional)

Star of the Meadow Lotion

This is a thick, rather heavy lotion, almost a cream. I've found it helpful for softening skin, particularly foot calluses and cracked cuticles.

It's a beautiful pale yellow, and without added fragrance, has a faint smell that's slightly carrot-like—a smell that fades over the course of a week or so.

The two main components are seed oils of meadowfoam—a wildflower—and borage—an herb also called starflower. Meadowfoam is a light oil, while borage is much heavier, so the proportions are adjusted to balance the two.

Oil Phase

34 grams (1.2 ounces) meadowfoam oil
9 grams (.3 ounce) borage oil
9 grams (.3 ounce) shea butter
9 grams (.3 ounce) stearic acid
23 grams (.8 ounce) emulsifying wax
6 grams (.2 ounce) vitamin E oil

Water Phase

360 grams (12.7 ounces) distilled water

Cool Down Phase

5 grams (.2 ounce) Germaben II or Optiphen
Up to 6 grams (.2 ounce) scent (optional)

Almond and Cocoa Butter Lotion

Almond oil has a silky feel I particularly like. Cocoa butter offers a little richness without oiliness. This lotion is light and creamy, and was a favorite among my testers.

Oil Phase

    48 grams (1.7 ounces) almond oil
    9 grams (.3 ounce) cocoa butter
    9 grams (.3 ounce) stearic acid
    23 grams (.8 ounce) emulsifying wax
    6 grams (.2 ounce) vitamin E oil

Water Phase

    354 grams (12.5 ounces) distilled water

Cool Down Phase

    5 grams (.2 ounce) Germaben II or Optiphen
    Up to 6 grams (.2 ounce) scent (optional)

Almond and Coconut Lotion

This is a very light lotion you might prefer in the summer or if you don't need much moisturizing.

Oil Phase

34 grams (1.2 ounces) almond oil
26 grams (.9 ounce) coconut oil
6 grams (.2 ounce) stearic acid
14 grams (.5 ounce) conditioning emulsifier
6 grams (.2 ounce) vitamin E oil

Water Phase

363 grams (12.8 ounces) distilled water

Cool Down Phase

5 grams (.2 ounce) Germaben II or Optiphen
Up to 6 grams (.2 ounce) scent (optional)

Autumn Lotion

Hazelnut oil and pumpkin seed butter make this lotion almost sound edible. Of course it's not—but it's a silky, medium-weight lotion that makes your skin feel smooth.

Oil Phase

71 grams (2.5 ounces) hazelnut oil
17 grams (.6 ounce) pumpkin seed butter
17 grams (.6 ounce) stearic acid
23 grams (.8 ounce) emulsifying wax
6 grams (.2 ounce) vitamin E oil

Water Phase

179 grams (6.3 ounces) distilled water
136 grams (4.8 ounces) aloe vera gel (See notes.)

Cool Down Phase

5 grams (.2 ounce) Germaben II or Optiphen
Up to 6 grams (.2 ounce) scent (optional)

Notes

Aloe vera gel, as sold by soapmaking and lotion suppliers, is actually a liquid. Don't confuse it with aloe vera gel that's sold as burn medication.

Rice Bran and Shea Lotion

Rice bran oil leaves very little oily feeling on the skin, so this is a light lotion, with just enough shea butter to make it richer.

Oil Phase

> 48 grams (1.7 ounces) rice bran oil
> 6 grams (.2 ounce) shea butter
> 14 grams (.5 ounce) stearic acid
> 23 grams (.8 ounce) emulsifying wax
> 6 grams (.2 ounce) vitamin E oil

Water Phase

> 351 grams (12.4 ounces) distilled water

Cool Down Phase

> 5 grams (.2 ounce) Germaben II or Optiphen
> Up to 6 grams (.2 ounce) scent (optional)

Hemp and Almond Lotion

Hemp oil is soothing and good for the skin. It also gives this lotion a faint smell of fresh rope that many people like.

Oil Phase

    30 grams (1.1 ounce) hemp oil
    30 grams (1.1 ounce) almond oil
    9 grams (.3 ounce) stearic acid
    23 grams (.8 ounce) emulsifying wax
    6 grams (.2 ounce) vitamin E oil

Water Phase

    351 grams (12.4 ounces) distilled water

Cool Down Phase

    5 grams (.2 ounce) Germaben II or Optiphen
    Up to 6 grams (.2 ounce) scent (optional) (See notes.)

Notes

If you want to add scent, make sure you choose one that complements the natural hemp smell. I'd suggest sweetgrass, sandalwood, patchouli, or musk. One friend liked star anise essential oil.

Shea, Silk, and Chamomile Lotion

This lotion feels very light going on, and leaves a silky after-feel. With its faint, pleasant scent of chamomile, it's a good choice for a lotion with no added scent.

Oil Phase

33 grams (1.2 ounces) jojoba oil
33 grams (1.2 ounces) shea oil
11 grams (.4 ounce) stearic acid
17 grams (.6 ounce) emulsifying wax
6 grams (.2 ounce) conditioning emulsifier
6 grams (.2 ounce) vitamin E oil

Water Phase

320 grams (11.3 ounces) chamomile tea (See notes.)
22 grams (.8 ounce) silk amino acids

Cool Down Phase

5 grams (.2 ounce) Germaben II or Optiphen
Up to 6 grams (.2 ounce) scent (optional)

Notes

Make the chamomile tea in advance with distilled water and either loose tea or bags. With loose tea, strain carefully.

Ingrid's Magic Potion Lotion

I took one look at Ingrid's long list of ingredients and wondered whether the lotion would really be worth the trouble and expense. After one try, I decided it was—at least for my skin. The lotion is slightly thinner than most, but still rich and emollient.

Oil Phase

   18 grams (.6 ounce) macadamia oil
   18 grams (.6 ounce) shea butter
   18 grams (.6 ounce) apricot kernel oil
   15 grams (.5 ounce) avocado oil
   9 grams (.3 ounce) rosehip oil
   9 grams (.3 ounce) evening primrose oil
   21 grams (.7 ounce) stearic acid
   21 grams (.7 ounce) emulsifying wax
   6 grams (.2 ounce) vitamin E oil

Water Phase

   318 grams (11.2 ounces) chamomile tea (See notes.)

Cool Down Phase

   5 grams (.2 ounce) green tea extract (optional)
   5 grams (.2 ounce) calendula extract (optional)
   5 grams (.2 ounce) spirulina extract (optional)
   5 grams (.2 ounce) Germaben II or Optiphen
   Up to 6 grams (.2 ounce) scent (optional)

Notes

Make the chamomile tea in advance with distilled water and either loose tea or bags. With loose tea, strain carefully. Make the tea perhaps a bit darker than if you were going to drink it. You can substitute green tea or rosehip water.

The extracts for the cool down phase are optional, but very good. The calendula has a light smell of its own.

For consistency with the other recipes in this book, I've added Germaben II as a choice of preservative, but Ingrid herself prefers Optiphen.

This lotion takes a little longer to set than most.

Suz's Light Lotion

This lotion is light, silky, and easy to make. Suz prefers it without glycerin, but she includes that ingredient as an option for friends who like it.

Oil Phase

   28 grams (1 ounce) fractionated coconut oil
   28 grams (1 ounce) almond oil
   3 grams (.1 ounce) glycerin (optional)
   10 grams (.4 ounce) stearic acid
   24 grams (.8 ounce) emulsifying wax
   6 grams (.2 ounce) vitamin E oil

Water Phase

   357 grams (12.6 ounces) distilled water

Cool Down Phase

   5 grams (.2 ounce) Germaben II or Optiphen
   Up to 6 grams (.2 ounce) scent (optional)

Milly's Body Lotion

This is a medium-rich lotion, not heavy. The mango butter is astringent, so the lotion may have the temporary effect of tightening the skin.

Oil Phase

14 grams (.5 ounce) sweet almond oil
10 grams (.4 ounce) mango butter
10 grams (.4 ounce) cocoa butter
9 grams (.3 ounce) jojoba oil
9 grams (.3 ounce) macadamia nut oil
25 grams (.9 ounce) emulsifying wax
5 grams (.2 ounce) vitamin E oil

Water Phase

375 grams (13.2 ounces) distilled water

Cool Down Phase

5 grams (.2 ounce) Germaben II or Optiphen
Up to 6 grams (.2 ounce) scent (optional)

Notes

Milly herself makes this without preservative. Of course, if you do that, you should use Pro Technique for sanitation.

Milk Lotion Recipes
Treating Your Skin to Milk

Milk helps make lotions that are rich but light, soothing but non-oily. They do require more care in sanitation, though, because of the greater likelihood of spoilage. Even if you make them only for yourself, you should use Pro Technique. Also, even with Pro Technique, use only milk that's pasteurized.

In these recipes, in place of Germaben II, I specify Germaben IIE, a preservative designed for higher-fat lotions. That's because milk products, while used as "water phase" ingredients, contribute a significant amount of fat.

Fermented milk products like buttermilk and yogurt contain skin-nourishing alpha hydroxy acids, but they may also contain active cultures. And active cultures, though excellent for digestion, are not a good thing at all in lotion. So, when buying such products for *lotion,* make sure the label does *not* say it contains active cultures—or else be extra careful to heat adequately when sanitizing. And definitely test the lotion for live organisms after it's made.

Linda's Goat Milk Lotion

Rich and soothing, this lotion was a favorite among the recipe testers for this book.

Oil Phase

    40 grams (1.4 ounces) almond oil
    27 grams (1 ounce) coconut oil
    13 grams (.5 ounce) apricot kernel oil
    13 grams (.5 ounce) pumpkin seed butter
    11 grams (.4 ounce) emulsifying wax
    11 grams (.4 ounce) conditioning emulsifier
    6 grams (.2 ounce) vitamin E oil

Water Phase

    333 grams (11.7 ounces) pasteurized goat milk

Cool Down Phase

    5 grams (.2 ounce) Germaben IIE or Optiphen
    Up to 6 grams (.2 ounce) scent (optional)

Notes

Because this recipe contains milk, you should use Pro Technique for proper sanitation.

Deena's Goat Milk Lotion

Goat milk, jojoba oil, aloe vera, and glycerin make this a rich, soothing lotion that's especially good in damp climates.

Oil Phase

> 147 grams (5.2 ounces) coconut oil
> 5 grams (.2 ounce) jojoba oil
> 9 grams (.3 ounce) stearic acid
> 18 grams (.6 ounce) emulsifying wax
> 5 grams (.2 ounce) vitamin E oil

Water Phase

> 151 grams (5.3 ounces) aloe vera gel (See notes.)
> 96 grams (3.4 ounces) pasteurized goat milk
> 18 grams (.6 ounce) glycerin

Cool Down Phase

> 5 grams (.2 ounce) Germaben IIE or Optiphen
> Up to 6 grams (.2 ounce) scent (optional)

Notes

Because this recipe contains milk, you should use Pro Technique for proper sanitation.

Aloe vera gel, as sold by soapmaking and lotion suppliers, is actually a liquid. Don't confuse it with aloe vera gel that's sold as burn medication.

When you combine the water phase ingredients, they will look curdled. Don't worry—they'll smooth out just fine as you stick blend the lotion.

Another "don't worry": This lotion takes longer to set than most. You might be afraid it won't set at all, but give it time.

Almond Milk and Pistachio Lotion

This gives you the rich, light, soothing lotion typical of a milk recipe, but without using animal products.

Oil Phase

    68 grams (2.4 ounces) pistachio oil
    11 grams (.4 ounce) stearic acid
    16 grams (.6 ounce) emulsifying wax
    7 grams (.2 ounce) conditioning emulsifier
    6 grams (.2 ounce) vitamin E oil

Water Phase

    349 grams (12.3 ounces) almond milk (See notes.)

Cool Down Phase

    5 grams (.2 ounce) Germaben IIE or Optiphen
    Up to 6 grams (.2 ounce) scent (optional)

Notes

Because this recipe contains nut milk, you should use Pro Technique for proper sanitation.

Almond oil may be substituted for pistachio. But pistachio sinks into the skin especially well, so it's worth obtaining.

Almond milk is made by pulverizing almonds, steeping in very hot water, and straining out the solids. Though you can buy "almond milk," the commercial product contains quite a few ingredients besides almonds and water and is *not* suitable for making lotion.

Here's how to make your own: In a countertop blender, blend about 2 ounces (about 50 grams) of almonds with about 3 cups (about .7 liter) of distilled water that has been heated near boiling—as if you were making tea. You can instead do this in a food processor, if yours is large enough to handle that much liquid without running over. Or simply grind or finely chop the almonds before adding to the water. Let the mixture stand about three minutes, then pour through a very fine strainer.

When sanitizing almond milk with Pro Technique, I put the whole amount I've made into the oven and then afterwards *remove* what I don't need. That makes the milk a bit richer than if I compensate for evaporation by adding distilled water. But either way is fine.

Goat Milk, Chamomile, and Jojoba Lotion

This recipe is good as is, but it's also meant to inspire your own formulations. The idea is that an herb can offer a lot to a lotion, and so can milk. By using dehydrated milk, you can have both. Just be sure your herb is one that, like chamomile, is skin-safe.

Oil Phase

> 31 grams (1.1 ounces) jojoba oil
> 31 grams (1.1 ounces) almond oil
> 9 grams (.3 ounce) shea butter
> 20 grams (.7 ounce) emulsifying wax
> 5 grams (.2 ounce) conditioning emulsifier
> 6 grams (.2 ounce) vitamin E oil

Water Phase

> 292 grams (10.3 ounces) chamomile tea (See notes.)
> 55 grams (1.9 ounces) powdered goat milk (See notes.)

Cool Down Phase

> 5 grams (.2 ounce) Germaben IIE or Optiphen
> Up to 6 grams (.2 ounce) scent (optional)

Notes

Because this recipe contains milk, you should use Pro Technique for proper sanitation.

Make the chamomile tea in advance with distilled water and either loose tea or bags. With loose tea, strain carefully.

When adding the powdered goat milk to the chamomile tea, stir to dissolve. You may need your stick blender to eliminate lumps.

Buttermilk, Hazelnut, and Honey Lotion

This recipe almost sounds like it's for a dessert, but it's really for something even better—a lotion that will make your skin feel wonderful.

Oil Phase

> 65 grams (2.3 ounces) hazelnut oil
> 5 grams (.2 ounce) cocoa butter
> 16 grams (.6 ounce) emulsifying wax
> 7 grams (.2 ounce) conditioning emulsifier
> 6 grams (.2 ounce) vitamin E oil

Water Phase

> 326 grams (11.5 ounces) reconstituted buttermilk
> (See notes.)
> 25 grams (.9 ounce) honeyquat (See notes.)

Cool Down Phase

> 5 grams (.2 ounce) Germaben IIE or Optiphen
> Up to 6 grams (.2 ounce) scent (optional)

Notes

Because this recipe contains buttermilk, you should use Pro Technique for proper sanitation.

For this recipe, I specify reconstituted buttermilk, as it's thinner and more predictable than regular buttermilk, and also less likely to contain active cultures. Make it from powder in accordance with manufacturer's directions.

Important: Make sure your buttermilk powder does not contain active cultures, or else be extra careful to heat adequately when sanitizing. And definitely test the lotion for live organisms after it's made.

Honeyquat is a derivative of honey. There are other honey derivatives that could be used instead, in accordance with manufacturer's directions.

Golden Lotion

The great majority of my recipes are simple, inexpensive, and reasonable in every way. But I couldn't resist—just once—loading a lotion with every wonderful ingredient on the shelf. The lotion is pale gold in color, but also "golden" in the sense that it's costlier to make than most of my recipes. (Which still doesn't put it, ounce for ounce, nearly in the price range of even an average commercial product!)

Is it worth the prime ingredients and the extra trouble? Like any lotion, it's worth it if it's right for *you*.

This is a soothing, non-greasy lotion that is softening and conditioning for your skin. For winter use in harsh climates, it might not be rich enough. The tamanu oil gives it a pleasant, faint smell like black walnuts.

Oil Phase

   30 grams (1.1 ounces) pistachio oil
   20 grams (.7 ounce) tamanu oil
   10 grams (.4 ounce) olive squalane
   10 grams (.4 ounce) aloe vera extract oil
   10 grams (.4 ounce) argan oil
   5 grams (.2 ounce) cupuaçu butter
   2 grams (.1 ounce) marula oil
   16 grams (.6 ounce) emulsifying wax
   7 grams (.2 ounce) conditioning emulsifier
   6 grams (.2 ounce) vitamin E oil

Water Phase

    225 grams (7.9 ounces) chamomile tea (See notes.)
    30 grams (1.1 ounces) powdered buttermilk (See notes.)
    25 grams (.9 ounce) honeyquat
    25 grams (.9 ounce) silk amino acids
    30 grams (1.1 ounces) aloe vera gel (See notes.)

Cool Down Phase

    5 grams (.2 ounce) Germaben IIE or Optiphen
    Up to 6 grams (.2 ounce) scent (optional)

Notes

Because this recipe contains buttermilk, you should use Pro Technique for proper sanitation.

Make the chamomile tea in advance with distilled water and either loose tea or bags. With loose tea, strain carefully.

When adding the powdered buttermilk to the chamomile tea, stir to dissolve. You may need your stick blender to eliminate lumps.

Important: Make sure your buttermilk powder does not contain active cultures, or else be extra careful to heat adequately when sanitizing. And definitely test the lotion for live organisms after it's made.

Aloe vera gel, as sold by soapmaking and lotion suppliers, is actually a liquid. Don't confuse it with aloe vera gel that's sold as burn medication.

Designing Your Own
How to Create Great Recipes

After you've made a few good lotions from my recipes, you'll probably be eager to branch out, try some modifications, and start formulating your own. This chapter will give you the background you need.

Ingredients

You'll control the kind of lotion you get by choosing the right fats, water-based liquids, emulsifiers, thickeners, and additives, and by adjusting the percentage of each.

Here's the basic framework for a lotion:

- Light oils—8% to 17%.
- Heavy oils or butters—up to 5%.
- Water or other liquids—75% to 80%.
- Emulsifying wax—3% to 6%. Or use another emulsifier at its recommended percentage.
- Thickener—up to 3%.
- Vitamin E oil—1%. Or use another antioxidant at its recommended percentage.
- Preservative—usually about 1%, but always follow manufacturer's directions.

We've already looked at the basic types of ingredients to see what goes into lotion. But now let's take a closer look, with an eye to designing recipes.

Fat

The oil phase ingredients in a lotion can be all oils, or a mixture of oils and butters. Following this chapter, you'll find a chart that rates many common fats for density, skin penetration, and oily feel. You can also judge this for yourself. Just try a little of the oil or butter on your hand to see how greasy it feels by itself. How long does it make your skin feel oily?

The lighter oils—the ones that penetrate skin well and have little oily residue—will be the main fat of most lotions. Some of the best for this are almond, jojoba, grapeseed, pistachio, sunflower, walnut, fractionated coconut, and hazelnut.

Butters and heavier oils are used in smaller amounts, the way a cook would use seasoning—a little goes a long way. They can contribute a lot to a lotion, but it's easy to overdo it, so add them cautiously. First try adding one at 1% to 2% of the total weight of your lotion. If it doesn't come out too heavy, use a little more of the fat in the next batch and compare the two.

Another important characteristic of fats is their smell. Those with distinctive natural smells include unrefined shea butter, cupuaçu butter, apricot kernel oil, argan oil, beeswax, hemp oil, virgin coconut oil, mango oil, unrefined jojoba oil, neem oil, unrefined wheat germ oil, tamanu oil, pumpkin seed butter, and unrefined cocoa butter. Some of these smells are subtle—others, such as those of neem and hemp, aren't subtle at all. Often a fat has a strong smell in its unrefined form, but less of one when refined.

If a lotion contains only a small amount of a strong-smelling fat, the smell will be very dilute and will probably fade before long. This would be true of most butters and quite a few oils—when you aren't using much, it's just not going to make a big difference. On the other hand, if that fat is a major ingredient, you'll have to take its smell into account.

The smell of some fats, such as tamanu oil and cocoa butter, is pleasant. The smells of unrefined shea butter, nut oils, beeswax, and cupuaçu butter are more neutral. Some people like the smell of hemp oil or neem, while others find them objectionable. Pleasant, neutral, and potentially unpleasant smells should all be considered in choosing fragrance or essential oils—some scents and some natural smells may go better together than others.

The natural smell of ingredients is especially important when you're making unscented lotions. People expect them not only to have no added scent, but to have no smell at all. For these lotions, you may prefer fats with little smell to start with, and in a refined form.

Mango butter and kokum butter are astringent, tightening the skin temporarily. This effect may work well in some lotions.

Mineral oil, a common ingredient in commercial lotions, is not a favorite among handcraft lotionmakers. I've experimented with light mineral oil and found it makes a fairly good lotion. However, it is much heavier—given the same percentages of thickener and emulsifier—than lotion made with plant oils. I did have one tester who preferred it to the lotions made with plant oils, saying it was good when massaging her cuticles.

Lotion made with silicone oils worked best for one of my testers—and not at all for some others. For most testers, though, they didn't seem to make any difference. Overall, I didn't find they improved my lotions, and they're not cheap. But you may be one of the people who prefer them, so you can experiment.

Water or Other Liquid

Distilled water works just fine for the water phase of lotion, but there are so many other possibilities! Different kinds of milk, hydrosols, aloe vera gel, herbal teas—and of course, you can combine them, too.

As with fats, be aware of the smell of your water phase ingredients. Some may have strong smells—as does, for example, undiluted evaporated milk.

If you're developing a recipe with milk, remember that part of your water phase is actually milk fat. If your lotion is turning out too thick or too oily, try increasing the percentage of water phase and decreasing the oil phase percentage. Or use lighter fats.

Only pasteurized milk should be used in lotion. Goat milk is popular among lotionmakers, but ordinary whole milk from cows works just as well.

Make sure that any herbal tea you use is skin-safe. Chamomile and calendula work well, but some other herbs might not.

Emulsifier

For decades, lotions and creams were made with beeswax and borax as the emulsifiers, with baking soda replacing borax in more recent times. These traditional ingredients can still be used successfully, especially with electric mixing tools such as stick blenders. However, they're more difficult to work with, and the emulsion is more likely to break down. I've admired lotion made by experts with these ingredients, but prefer others for my own use.

Many new emulsifiers have now been developed, and no doubt more are to come. Choosing among them is partly a matter of taste: What kind of texture do you want? Are you comfortable with processed emulsifiers? Or do you want a product that's more or less natural? Whatever product you choose, use it exactly as the manufacturer recommends!

Some emulsifiers have more than one component and must be mixed and balanced for the individual recipe. The emulsifiers I recommend, though—called *self emulsifiers*—are self-contained. They're much simpler to use and don't require complex calculations. There are many, many kinds available. I've used two in this book—emulsifying wax and conditioning emulsifier.

Emulsifying wax, or e-wax, will give your lotion more body. Added at the maximum percentage recommended by the manufacturer, it may leave a waxy after-feel. With lower percentages, you get a medium or light lotion, depending on your choice of fats.

Conditioning emulsifier may be called BTMS, or BTMS-25, or BTMS-50, or another name altogether. Used alone, it produces a very light lotion that feels almost watery as you rub it in. After that, the lotion seems to disappear—but it's very effective as a skin softener and conditioner.

For many recipes, I use two-thirds emulsifying wax and one-third conditioning emulsifier. For others, I use just one emulsifier but add a thickener.

Thickener

Stearic acid is one of the most popular thickeners for handcraft lotion. Others include cetyl alcohol, xanthan gum, and grain-based thickeners.

Follow the manufacturer's directions, if any. They should give you a range of percentages for thinner to thicker lotion.

You can also omit thickener entirely—if you do, you'll generally need more emulsifier.

Antioxidant

Common antioxidants include Vitamin E oil and rosemary extract. Don't mistake antioxidants for preservatives—they're not the same thing. Antioxidants stop fats from going rancid, while preservatives eliminate bacteria and molds.

Preservative

This has to be the most controversial topic in lotionmaking, hands down. There are those who would never make lotion with a preservative—at least, an artificial one—and those who would never make it *without* one. Also, individual preservatives have fans and attackers. It's a fraught subject.

I'd like to avoid taking sides but still set down a few guidelines. First, for those who will use commercial preservative:

• Use it only according to manufacturer's directions. Note the recommended percentages and temperature for its use.

• For lotion, you can normally use a preservative meant only for oil-in-water emulsions. But if you're making lotion with milk, you don't know the exact percentage of fat in the recipe. For these lotions, choose a preservative that works for both oil-in-water and water-in-oil emulsions.

For those who choose not to use preservative:

• Make your lotion with Pro Technique, as described in this book.

• Refrigerate your lotion, and discard it after a week to ten days.

• If you're selling your lotion, know the legal and insurance requirements.

Finally, for those considering a natural alternative:

• Research your alternative and decide whether it's safe and effective on the basis of scientific evidence from accredited sources. If it can't pass a laboratory challenge test, then it can't substitute for a commercial preservative!

Additives

The number of lotion additives available, for both practical and aesthetic purposes, is beyond anyone's guess. Some are herbal, some artificial.

Glycerin is a popular additive, but it works better in damp climates than in dry. It attracts water to itself, which is fine when that water is pulled from the air to moisturize the skin. But if there's little water in the air, glycerin pulls water from the skin instead!

Silk amino acids—also called silk protein—add a desirable silky feeling to lotion.

Some lotionmakers add citric acid to adjust the lotion pH to the pH of the skin, or to the level a preservative requires.

Honey is less successful as an additive—it's undoubtedly good for skin, but it's sticky, even in small amounts. But honeyquat, which is manufactured from honey, is not sticky. It still retains a slight honey smell and is considered moisturizing. There are other honey derivatives as well.

Evaluate potential additives by researching them as much as you can. Then make two batches of the same lotion, one with the additive and one without. See whether there's actually any difference.

Many additives come with health claims, made directly or indirectly. Whether it's making age spots and scars fade, rejuvenating skin, curing eczema and psoriasis, or one of a host of other benefits, you can find an additive said to achieve it. And maybe some do, at least for some users.

But if you're selling lotion, this is risky territory. Making any claim of health benefits can reclassify your lotion as a drug. Even if you say it in a roundabout way, like, "This ingredient is believed to . . . ," you're not off the hook. And the legal requirements for drug approval are far beyond what most handcraft lotionmakers could possibly meet.

Controlling Consistency

Thickness and consistency of lotion are very important to most users. The problem is, not everyone wants the same thing. For some, a lotion's ability to sink into skin quickly without an oily residue is most important. Others prefer a creamier lotion.

Though we've already discussed some of this, here is a collection of guidelines for controlling consistency:

• Balance the fats, using more or less of the heavy oils and butters, depending on the desired creaminess or lightness.

• Choose an emulsifier that will give the consistency you want. If you're using both emulsifying wax and conditioning emulsifier, adjust the balance between them. Also, adjust the overall amount of emulsifier.

• Adjust the amounts of water phase ingredients like goat milk or silk amino acids that affect consistency and texture.

• Adjust the amount of thickener.

If you're formulating for yourself, you'll probably need to experiment a little to find out what feels ideal to you.

If you're selling lotion, you'll probably want to offer a variety of consistencies. Label them clearly, and maybe have tester bottles on hand.

Experimenting

Experimenting is the way to fine-tune your formulations and make them as good as they can be. Even "failures" are successes, because when something doesn't turn out, you find out what you can't do.

Write down everything you try. This will help you learn what works and what doesn't, and to repeat what works especially well. And of course, the first time you try anything, make a small batch. If you don't like it, you won't have lost much.

Test a new lotion for more than one use. A lotion too heavy for your hands might be perfect for feet or elbows. When you run out of that "too heavy" lotion, you may just decide to make more!

When trying out a new ingredient, add it to a formulation cautiously, starting with small amounts. See whether the difference in your lotion—if there is one—is something you want more of. A manufactured product will probably have a recommended range for its percentage in the lotion, and you can start low in that range. Also, check whether the new ingredient affects the type and amount of preservative you need.

To test any new ingredient seriously, make two batches of lotion, one with the ingredient and one without. Label the bottles with numbers only and give them to testers. If the new ingredient gets positive comments, weigh them against the effort and expense of adding the ingredient.

You may be surprised at the results. Lotionmakers may rave about the rare, newly discovered butter from the seeds of pink bananas, but that doesn't make pink banana seed butter any better than a more common fat available everywhere at a much lower price.

This book's recipe for Almond and Cocoa Butter Lotion provides a good example. Originally, my two primary ingredients for this recipe were almond oil and cupuaçu butter—an ingredient *du jour*. The lotion was excellent. Then it occurred to me that cupuaçu is a close relative of cacao, the tree that gives us chocolate. So, I made two lotions, identical except that one was 2% cupuaçu butter and the other was 2% cocoa butter. I sent the lotions, identified only by numbers, to my testers. They preferred the one with cocoa butter.

Remember: When you're experimenting, the only thing you're guaranteed to get is information!

Properties of Fats

	Density	Penetration	Oily Feel
Almond oil	Medium	Medium	Light
Apricot kernel oil	Light	Medium	Heavy
Avocado oil	Heavy	Poor	Heavy
Babassu oil	Solid	Good	Light
Borage seed oil	Medium	Good	Moderate
Castor oil	Heavy	Poor	Heavy
Cherry kernel oil	Medium	Medium	Light
Cocoa butter	Heavy	Poor	Heavy
Coconut oil	Heavy	Poor	Heavy
Coconut oil, fractionated	Light	Good	Minimal
Evening primrose oil	Light	Good	Light
Grapeseed oil	Light	Good	Light
Hazelnut oil	Light	Good	Light
Hemp oil	Medium	Poor	Medium
Illipe butter	Heavy	Poor	Heavy
Jojoba oil	Medium	Good	Minimal
Kukui nut oil	Light	Good	Minimal
Lanolin	Heavy	Poor	Heavy
Macadamia nut oil	Heavy	Poor	Heavy
Mango butter	Heavy	Medium	Light
Meadowfoam seed oil	Medium	Good	Minimal
Mineral oil, light	Light	Poor	Heavy

	Density	Penetration	Oily Feel
Olive oil	Heavy	Poor	Heavy
Olive squalane	Light	Good	Minimal
Palm oil	Heavy	Medium	Poor
Peach kernel oil	Light	Good	Minimal
Pecan oil	Medium	Good	Moderate
Pistachio oil	Light	Good	Minimal
Pomegranate seed oil	Medium	Good	Minimal
Pumpkin seed oil	Medium	Good	Light
Rice bran oil	Medium	Medium	Minimal
Rosehip oil	Medium	Medium	Moderate
Sal butter	Hard	Good	Moderate
Sesame oil	Heavy	Poor	Heavy
Shea butter	Heavy	Medium	Heavy
Shea oil	Medium	Medium	Moderate
Sunflower oil	Light	Good	Minimal
Tamanu oil	Light	Good	Minimal
Walnut oil	Medium	Good	Moderate
Wheat germ oil	Heavy	Poor	Heavy

Troubleshooting
Tricks, Tweaks, and Fixes

Lotions rarely fail, in the sense of being unusable. But maybe you didn't get what you wanted. You usually can't change a lotion once it's made, but you can adjust your recipe or methods for the next batch. These suggestions may help.

If your lotion is too thick . . .

• Decrease the amount of butters or heavy oils and increase the amount of light oils.

• Increase the amount of the water phase ingredient(s).

• If the recipe includes stearic acid or other thickener, decrease the amount or eliminate it completely. (You may then need more emulsifier.)

• Decrease the amount of emulsifying wax and increase the amount of conditioning emulsifier, keeping the total amount of emulsifier the same.

• If you like the lotion but don't like the way it dispenses from a regular bottle, put it in tottles.

If your lotion is too thin . . .

• Increase the amount of butters or heavy oils and decrease the amount of light oils.

• Decrease the amount of the water phase ingredient(s).

• Use up to 3% stearic acid or other thickener.

- Increase the amount of emulsifying wax and decrease the amount of conditioning emulsifier, keeping the total amount of emulsifier the same.
- Mix more thoroughly.

If your lotion feels greasy or waxy . . .

- Apply less lotion and give it a couple of minutes to sink in. Most of us are used to watery commercial lotions. Hand-crafted lotions may feel different from what you at first expect—though if you use them properly, they're much better for your skin.
- Substitute more easily absorbed oils and butters for those in the recipe. (Unlike in soapmaking, substituting ingredients doesn't make you revise your entire formulation.)
- If your lotion is milk-based, the fats in the milk may be giving you too high an overall percentage of fat. Try decreasing the amount of the oil phase ingredients and increasing the amount of the water phase ones.
- Decrease the amount of emulsifying wax and increase the amount of conditioning emulsifier, keeping the total amount of emulsifier the same.

If your lotion feels watery . . .

- Increase the amount of emulsifying wax and decrease the percentage of conditioning emulsifier, keeping the total emulsifier content the same.
- Decrease the total amount of the water phase.
- Use up to 3% stearic acid or other thickener.

If your lotion (or your skin) doesn't feel smooth . . .

• Substitute silky feeling oils such as almond oil for some of the oil phase content.

• Substitute silk amino acids for part of the water phase content.

• If your climate is reasonably humid, substitute glycerin for part of the water phase content.

• If the recipe includes stearic acid or other thickener, decrease the amount or eliminate it completely. (You may then need more emulsifier.)

• Decrease the amount of emulsifying wax and increase the amount of conditioning emulsifier, keeping the total amount of emulsifier the same.

If it separates or has a layer of water or oil . . .

• Mix more thoroughly.

• Check your recipe to make sure water and oil phase ingredients are within the percentage ranges given in the chapter on designing your own lotions.

• Increase the amount of emulsifier.

If there's a foam layer on top . . .

• Make sure the head of your stick blender is completely submerged in the lotion while you're using it.

• Stick blend less, stir more.

• As you bottle the lotion, pour against the side instead of squirting toward the bottom.

Making It a Business
How to Go Pro, Not Bust

If you're making lotion commercially, it's not enough to make great lotion. Among other things, you'll need commercial equipment, knowledge of legal requirements, and insurance. Here are a few pointers about lotionmaking as a business.

Commercial Equipment

You'll probably need more equipment to make lotion commercially, including larger containers for heating and mixing, and better bottling equipment.

If you're not quite ready to buy factory or laboratory equipment for thousands of dollars, see what's available for restaurants. A small restaurant would buy equipment at about the same level of expense as a small lotion business, and the sanitation needs are similar. You may find just the kind of mid-level equipment you need. For example, you could buy an industrial bottling machine, but why not first look into restaurant condiment pumps?

Not only might such equipment suit you better, but it might make some insurance companies less nervous about insuring you. Industrial equipment suggests large-scale production, which could mean greater risk of claims.

Regulations

Thoroughly research the safety and labeling regulations that govern cosmetics for sale in your jurisdiction. A full discussion of these rules is far beyond the scope of this book, so consult the Web sites and the available literature of official regulatory agencies. To get you started, you might also get help from professional organizations like the Handcrafted Soapmakers Guild in the United States, and the Guild of Craft Soap and Toiletry Makers in the United Kingdom.

In the United States, each state has its own regulations for cosmetics. Beyond that, cosmetics are regulated by the U.S. Food and Drug Administration (FDA), for any product involved in interstate commerce.

Now, before you sigh in relief because you have no plans to sell out of state, understand that "interstate commerce" covers a lot more than that. To avoid the classification, you'd also have to buy all your ingredients and packaging within your state. Plus there's a general consideration that anything you sell may be carried to another state after its purchase. So, almost regardless of your situation, you're stuck with following federal regulations.

A key term in FDA regulations is *adulterated*. This means that the cosmetic is contaminated, or includes substances that aren't approved, or simply isn't produced in a sanitary way. To make sure your lotion would not be considered adulterated or "potentially adulterated," follow the FDA Good Manufacturing Practice Guidelines. Of course, as we discussed earlier, you must also test your lotion.

Another key FDA term is *misbranded*. This means the maker didn't follow regulations for labeling. Any lotion that's sold must have a label, and it must include the same information whether you're making lotion by the pound or by the ton. The surprising thing is that many major U.S. manufacturers regularly flout these regulations. But whether *you* could get away with it is anybody's guess.

FDA regulations for cosmetics labeling go into great detail, including what you must include, what you must *not* include, order of information, directions to be given, warnings to be offered, font size, and location on the package. Ingredients must be listed with standard names from the International Nomenclature of Cosmetic Ingredients (INCI).

To avoid picking your own way through the officialese of U.S. labeling regulations, I highly recommend getting the book *Soap and Cosmetic Labeling,* by Marie Gale. This book explains federal regulations in easy-to-understand language with illustrations, and also gives links to state regulatory agencies.

The regulations we're discussing here are strictly for *cosmetics*. If you claim your lotion can cure, relieve, or treat a disease, that makes it a *drug*. This opens a whole new level of requirements for testing, and few handcraft lotionmakers would want to go there.

In case you wonder, you don't need any official certification to make and sell cosmetics in the United States, though many other countries require that.

In Canada, you must meet the standards for ingredients and labeling set by Health Canada, and also notify it of your intent to sell cosmetics.

In the European Union, products must be tested and certified for safety before they're sold. Labels must include even more information than in the United States, including identification of the individual batch number. The regulations in individual countries are supposed to follow the European Commission's Cosmetics Directive.

In Australia, lotionmakers must meet the requirements of the National Industrial Chemicals Notification and Assessment Scheme (NICNAS) and register with the agency. The regulations are similar to those of the FDA. Another agency that regulates cosmetics in that country is the Australian Competition and Consumer Commission (ACCC).

New Zealand has a Cosmetic Products Group Standard, which is based on Europe's Cosmetics Directive.

Insurance

Before you sell lotion, you should seriously consider getting insurance.

It's true that cases of people being harmed by lotion are very rare—the main exception involving lotion made for use near the eyes. As long as you're making lotion for the hands or body, the chances of a successful claim are small.

But even so, what would an *un*successful claim cost you? And what might it cost a store or craft fair where your lotion is sold? As protection against even unjust claims, insurance is very, very advisable.

Insurance companies vary in their approach toward handcraft lotionmakers. Some are very cautious, while others have found the risk of loss to be small, even with preservative-free lotion.

Research what's available to you, either directly or through professional associations. Look at the cost, but also consider other factors. Does the insurance cover you even if you're proven negligent? Does it have workspace requirements that are practical for you?

Those are questions to ask an insurer. Here are some that the insurer might ask you:

• Are your products all handmade? Handmade products mean smaller batch size, which limits the company's exposure to risk. The aim of this question isn't to make you use a stirring spoon instead of a stick blender—it's to weed out heavy manufacturing.

• Are any of your products legally considered drugs? Are any in a high-risk category?

• Have there ever been legal actions against you? If so, how were they settled?

• Do your labels meet government regulations?

• Are your suppliers and distributors added to your insurance through your agreements with them?

• Do you get warranties from your suppliers?

• Are your products tested?

• Do you have a *protocol* for sanitizing? This is a written procedure you follow each time you make lotion. It provides assurance that any problems with your lotion are not due to your own negligence.

Why, Why, Why?
Frequently Asked Questions

Why do your recipes make such small batches?

For personal use, a batch of that size is probably as much as you want to make at one time. And if you're making lotion for sale, it's best to make a small test batch with any formulation to see whether you like the lotion.

How do I increase the batch size?

Each of the recipes in the book will make about one pound of lotion. So, just multiply the amount of each ingredient by the number of pounds of lotion you want.

My methods aren't intended for mass production, but I have tripled a recipe size with good results. For large quantities, you might want to add the water phase a little more slowly to the oil phase to make sure all the ingredients combine well.

How do I substitute ingredients for the ones in your recipes?

You can experiment with ingredients as long as you stick to the basic structure of a lotion formulation. See the chapter on designing your own lotions.

I can't get goat milk. Is cow milk OK?

If you substitute cow milk for goat in a recipe and want to minimize the change, use whole milk. It has about the same butterfat content as commercial goat milk.

Why don't any of your recipes use silicone oils?

I like silicone oils in creams, but not in lotions—and my recipes don't include anything I've found disappointing. But silicone oils may work better for you. Feel free to try what appeals to you!

Why don't your recipes use natural emulsifiers or natural preservatives?

Most of the natural emulsifier recipes I've seen are for creams, not lotions. My efforts to reformulate for a lighter product were disastrous. Though I can't say it's impossible to use natural emulsifiers for lotion, it would clearly be an approach all its own, and beyond the scope of this book.

As for natural preservatives, the available information is so contradictory, and the subject is so controversial, I decided to stay out of the fray. Also, different countries have adopted different policies about natural preservatives, making it difficult to recommend anything in a book meant to be read internationally.

But what I *will* say is this: Research *any* preservative you're considering, using information sources that are independent from sales promotion. Look at legal and insurance issues, effectiveness and allergy risk, and decide for yourself if the product meets your needs.

Why don't you use [my other favorite lotion ingredient]? Don't you know it's the most wonderful ever?

Space and time didn't let me include everything that might work in lotion. Many proprietary ingredients come and go on the market so quickly that any book containing them would become outdated. Some ingredients are not legally accepted everywhere, or not available everywhere. Some are controversial. Some are hyped, overrated, and overpriced. For all those reasons, I mostly stuck to the basics.

But I hope you'll use my techniques to experiment with any ingredient that appeals to you. If you do experiment, be careful to follow a manufacturer's directions and comply with any applicable laws.

If alcohol is a good sanitizer, why use only 70%? Why not higher, like 92% or 99%? Stronger is better, right?

You might think the stronger alcohol used for degreasing electronics is better because it's stronger. It isn't better—it evaporates too quickly to sanitize reliably.

I have a dishwasher with a sanitizing cycle. Can I use that to sanitize my bottles and equipment?

I don't recommend it. It's not reliable, because it depends on the temperature of the water coming into it. Also, you can't use it for bottles, because the water spray won't do a good job of getting through the narrow necks. Plus, the heat may be too high for some plastic bottles and tops.

If you're selling lotion, you need to be able to defend your method, if you're ever challenged. You can't do that if you're sanitizing in the dishwasher, because it's not practical to verify the water temperature.

When you sanitize your bottles and equipment the night before, won't they just get recontaminated?

No. It's often done this way in laboratories. Turn the containers upside down, set the bottles on a bottle tree, and cover any flat tools such as spoons with plastic wrap. I've actually had a bottle tested that had been sanitized and left on a bottle tree for days. It was sanitary.

Why weigh the water? Why not just use a measuring cup?

Personally, I think it's easier to weigh. But for water, you *can* use a measuring cup, because—*only* for water—fluid ounces and weight ounces are the same. For anything else, measuring by volume won't give you accurate quantities.

How do I figure how much scent to add?

The amount depends on how much you like. And some scents are stronger than others. Also, the strength of a fragrance or essential oil of the same name can vary among vendors. Scents may also change once they're on your skin. Check the vendor's recommendations, if any, then add cautiously.

Are scents affected by lotionmaking? Is it like cold process soapmaking, which turns vanilla brown and makes citrus essential oils vanish?

In my experience, scents are unchanged in lotionmaking. I've never had vanilla go brown, or had any scent vanish or change.

Why do you prefer mason jars for weighing and heating?

Mason jars have advantages over anything else I've tried. They're cheap and easily available. They're heat resistant for both oven and microwave. Their lids are uniform and replaceable, and tight enough to prevent most evaporation of water phase ingredients during sanitization. And there are funnels made specially to fit the jars.

Any mason jar is fine, but I prefer the so-called "mason jar mugs," because I like the handles. With those, get the ones that are heat-treated.

What else besides mason jars works for Pro Technique?

You could heat your ingredients in the microwave in Pyrex measuring pitchers, tightly covered with plastic wrap. Then, for sanitizing, either replace the plastic wrap with aluminum foil or silicone lids, or transfer the ingredients to ovenproof casseroles, saucepans, or other containers. Be sure to correct the weight of the water phase after sanitizing, because you'll get more evaporation.

I read that germs can live only in water. Why do you sanitize fats in the oven?

One or another kind of bacteria or mold can survive just about anywhere.

To kill germs, why don't you just heat till the water phase ingredients come to a boil?

It's good enough to bring everything to 180°F (about 80°C). Boiling would greatly increase water evaporation. Also, heating to the boiling point of water can damage some fats and other ingredients, especially milk.

Why do you use a separate container for mixing? Can't you stick blend your lotion in one of the heating containers?

You could. Since I use glass heating containers, I don't. I'm afraid they'll break. Also, I find hot containers unpleasant to handle.

Why use a stick blender? Why not just stir with a spoon?

Lotion can be mixed by hand, but it's slower, and you have to be very thorough or it can set inconsistently—thicker in some bottles, thinner in others.

Can I use a cookie press, frosting gun, or something similar to fill bottles?

What you have is about sixteen ounces of hot liquid—more, if you've increased my recipe size—that's quickly developing the consistency of mayonnaise. You're racing to get it into bottles before it does.

There really aren't any special devices made for this, so you can try anything you think might work. Whatever it is, it should be quick and easy to use, and easy to wash and sanitize.

In the few years since I first wrote on soapmaking, I've seen improvements in the equipment available to handcraft soapmakers. As lotionmaking becomes more popular, maybe the same thing will happen. Meanwhile, we'll have to keep using and adapting cooking tools, restaurant equipment, and lab ware. Use your ingenuity—maybe *you'll* invent the perfect tools for smart lotionmaking!

Help! I keep forgetting to add the scent or the preservative!

Try putting them in the bottling area instead of the mixing area. You won't forget if they're right beside your empty bottles.

Help! My lotion didn't thicken!

Don't give up until you've waited at least 24 hours. Many lotions remain liquid for quite a while.

If there's no improvement, the chapter on troubleshooting can help you adjust your recipe or method for next time. But you can also save a too-thin batch, by using what I call a *cold emulsifier*—an emulsifier that can be added after the fact, at room temperature. These products have various names, but many vendors sell them. If you experiment much with your lotion recipes, it's not a bad idea to have one of these on hand.

When big companies make lotion, are their procedures the same as yours, only scaled up?

I posed this question to a biochemist specializing in commercial cosmetic formulation. He told me the procedures of a commercial cosmetics company were basically the same, with two differences: (1) Instead of a blender, they'd use a homogenizer, for a much finer, more stable emulsion. (2) Added scents were coupled with emulsifiers of their own.

Both of these, he said, helped keep the emulsion stable for twelve months, which is the time those companies must allow for distribution and adequate shelf life.

If what you say about U.S. labeling regulations is correct, even big companies are breaking the law! Why shouldn't I do that, too?

This is a tough question, and I don't have an answer. The laws are on the books, and they're not being enforced uniformly. This means you might get away with "misbranding," and then again, you might not. I wouldn't risk it.

Resources

Where to Read More

Soap & Cosmetic Labeling: How to Follow the Rules and Regs Explained in Plain English, Second Edition, by Marie Gale, Cinnabar Press, Broadbent, Oregon, 2010.

Microbial Quality Assurance in Cosmetics, Toiletries, and Non-Sterile Pharmaceuticals, Second Edition, edited by R. M. Baird with S. F. Bloomfield, Taylor & Francis/CRC Press, London and Bristol, Pennsylvania, 1996. Often listed as **Microbial Quality Assurance in Pharmaceuticals, Cosmetics, and Toiletries.**

Where to Get Testing

The following testers are all in the United States. For other countries, try searching online for "cosmetic testing lab," or contact your regional soapmaking guild.

Adamson Analytical Laboratories

www.adamsonlab.com

Marypaul Laboratories

www.marypaullabs.com

Sagescript Institute

www.sagescript.com

Where to Get Supplies

Most soapmaking supply Web sites offer many of the same ingredients lotionmakers use. Other suppliers cater especially to lotionmaking. I can't catalog them all, but here are a few that I've used and found helpful, or that have been recommended.

United States

Bramble Berry

Oils and butters, fragrance and essential oils, emulsifiers, cold emulsifier, bottles, miscellaneous lotion supplies.

www.brambleberry.com

Kangaroo Blue

Oils and butters, additives, containers.

www.kangarooblue.com

Lotioncrafter

Everything lotion, including hard-to-find ingredients and equipment.

www.lotioncrafter.com

Majestic Mountain Sage

Oils and butters, fragrance and essential oils, emulsifiers, cold emulsifier, bottles, miscellaneous lotion supplies.

www.thesage.com

Old Will Knott Scales

Inexpensive scales that read in both ounces and grams.

www.oldwillknottscales.com

Oregon Trail Soap Supplies & More

Oils and butters, fragrance and essential oils, cold emulsifier.

www.oregontrailsoaps.com

SKS Bottles and Packaging

Every kind of bottle and jar you can imagine.

www.sks-bottle.com

Soaper's Choice (Columbus Foods)

Oils and butters in larger quantities at lower prices.

www.soaperschoice.com

Wholesale Supplies Plus

Oils and butters, fragrance and essential oils, bottles.

www.wholesalesuppliesplus.com

Canada

Lynden House International

Oils and butters, fragrance and essential oils, additives, bottles.

www.lyndenhouse.net

Saffire Blue Inc.

Oils and butters, additives, cold emulsifier, bottles, equipment.

www.saffireblue.ca

United Kingdom

Gracefruit

Essential and fragrance oils, butters and oils, additives, organic products, bottles.

www.gracefruit.com

The Soap Kitchen

Oils and butters, additives, cold emulsifier, bottles, equipment.

www.thesoapkitchen.co.uk

Summer Naturals

Oils and butters, essential oils, bottles.

www.summernaturals.co.uk

Australia

Aussie Soap Supplies

Fragrance and essential oils, oils and butters, additives.

www.aussiesoapsupplies.com.au

Escentials of Australia

Oils and butters, fragrance and essential oils, additives, bottles.

www.escentialsofaustralia.com

New Directions Australia

Essential oils, additives, bottles.

www.newdirections.com.au

Index

About the Author

Anne L. Watson is the first author to have introduced modern techniques of home soapmaking and lotionmaking to book readers. She has made soap under the company name Soap Tree, and before her retirement from professional life, she was a historic preservation architecture consultant.

Besides her soap and lotion books, Anne has written practical guides to such topics as cookie molds and housekeeping, along with a number of literary novels. She and her husband, Aaron Shepard, live in Friday Harbor, Washington. You can visit her at

www.annelwatson.com

CPSIA information can be obtained
at www.ICGtesting.com
Printed in the USA
LVOW04s2259160217

524580LV00018B/175/P

9 781620 355138